MAIN DISEASES IN POULTRY FARMING
BACTERIAL INFECTIONS

For this English edition:

Main diseases in poultry farming. Bacterial infections

Plaza Antonio Beltrán Martínez nº 1, planta 8 - letra I
(Centro empresarial El Trovador)
50002 Zaragoza - Spain

First printing: december 2016

ISBN: 978-84-16818-39-6
D.L.: Z 1559-2016

Design, layout and printing:
Servet editorial - Grupo Asís Biomedia, S.L.
www.grupoasis.com
info@grupoasis.com

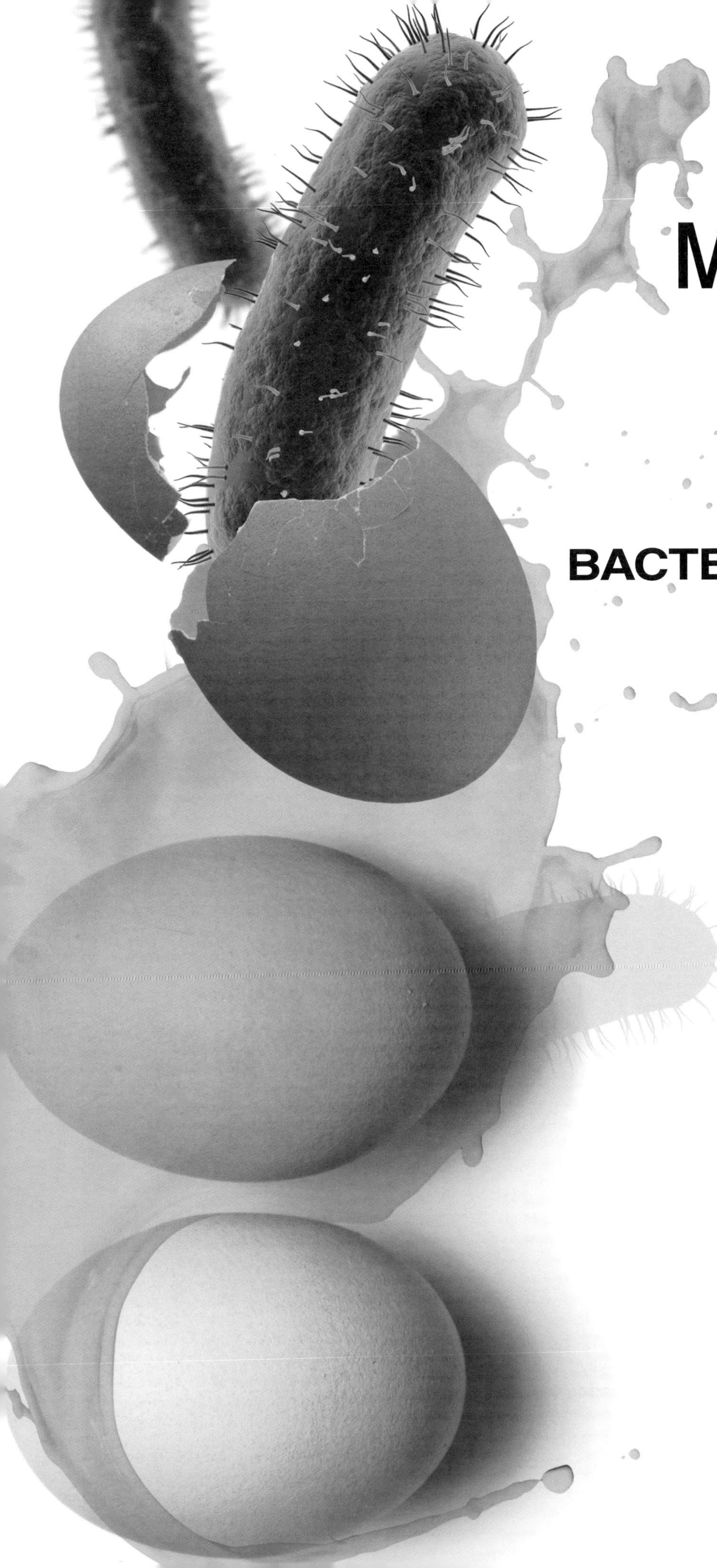

Main diseases in poultry farming

BACTERIAL INFECTIONS

Hafez Mohamed Hafez
Rüdiger Hauck

SERVET

ACKNOWLEDGEMENTS

We would like to thank all our colleagues who encouraged us in writing this book. We are especially grateful to those colleagues who generously let us use their excellent pictures, which make this book special. We also want to thank the publishing team for making this high-quality book possible. We hope it will be of value to veterinarians and other professionals interested in poultry diseases.

AUTHORS

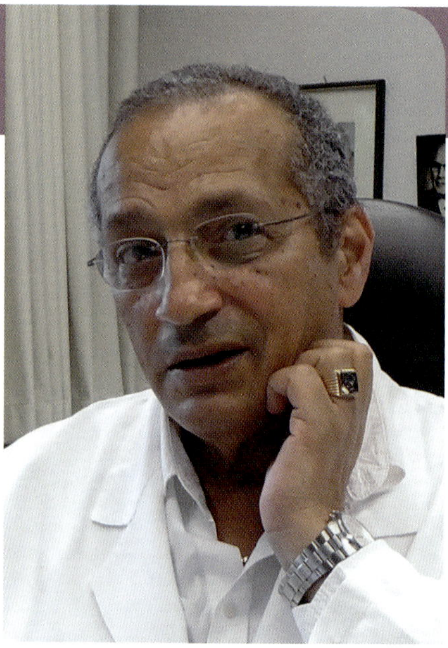

Hafez Mohamed Hafez

Prof. Dr. Dr. Hafez is a head of the Institute of Poultry Diseases at the Free University of Berlin. He gained his Master of Veterinary Science (MVSc) at the department of Poultry Diseases from Cairo University in 1975, and completed his Dr. medicinae veterinariae (Dr. med. vet.) at the department of Poultry Diseases, Giessen University, Germany in 1981. He finished the Dr. habilitatus (Dr. med. vet. habil.) thesis at the department of Poultry Diseases, Munich University, Germany in 1994.

Dr. Hafez is Veterinary Poultry Specialist since 1982, Veterinary Microbiology Specialist since 1989, Veterinary Animal Hygiene Specialist since 1996, Diplomate of European College of Veterinary Public Health (Dipl. ECVPH) since 2005, and Diplomate of European College of Poultry Veterinary Science (Dipl. ECPVS) since 2009. Dr. Hafez's career has focused on poultry diseases diagnosis and control in general and in particular respiratory and foodborne diseases, management, and hygiene. He is currently the Honorary Life President of the World Veterinary Poultry Association (WVPA). He is Past-President of the WVPA, Past-President of ECPVS, Chairman of Poultry Scientific Committee of the German Veterinary Chamber, Chairman of the German Branch of the World Veterinary Poultry Association and Chairman Working group 10 (Turkey) of the European Branch of World Poultry Science Association (WPSA). In addition, he is an honour Professor at the University of Hohenheim since 1996 as well as honour Professor at the Alexandria University, Egypt since 2009. Since 2015 he is advisor of the Arab Federation for Food Industries (AFFI). Furthermore, he is a member of several other scientific committees related to veterinary medicine. He is author and co-author of 231 articles in peer-reviewed journals and 49 book chapters.

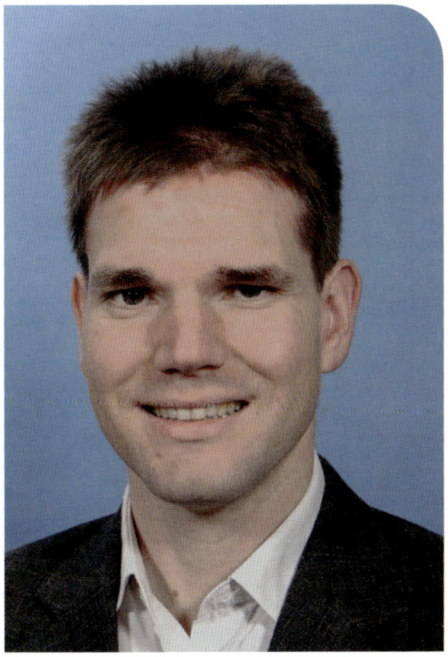

Rüdiger Hauck

Dr. Rüdiger Hauck is Research Scholar at the School of Veterinary Medicine, University of California, Davis (USA), where he does research on the causative viruses of avian influenza, avian encephalomyelitis and infectious bronchitis. He received his degree in Veterinary Sciences from Free University of Berlin in 2002. He completed his Dr. medicinae veterinariae (Dr. med. vet.) at the Institute for Poultry Diseases of the Free University of Berlin in 2006. He is Certified Veterinary Specialist for Poultry Diseases and Microbiology and Diplomate of the European College of Poultry Veterinary Science (ECPVS). His areas of interest include viral vaccination studies, detection and typing of bacterial pathogens, and studies of protozoan parasites. Dr. Hauck worked as Veterinary Consultant at the Bundesamt für Verbraucherschutz und Lebensmittelsicherheit (Federal Office of Consumer Protection and Food Safety), where he was a member of the team Antimicrobial Resistance. He is co-author of 41 articles in peer-reviewed journals and three book chapters.

FOREWORD

Bacterial diseases are a significant economic constraint on poultry production all over the world. Bacteria can cause serious diseases and could be a primary or secondary cause of disease. In addition, several of the bacteria that infect poultry have zoonotic potential including some of the bacteria involved in human food safety. Some members of that group infect and replicate efficiently in poultry without causing overt signs of disease, but once transmitted to humans could cause disease.

Advances in biology including molecular biology have been highly useful in understanding several facets of bacterial diseases including the pathogenesis, epidemiology, diagnosis, and control of bacterial diseases of poultry. With the rapid pace of change, it becomes essential to have new publications containing these new developments. This book reflects that need and provides updated and concise information on bacterial diseases of poultry. It is highly useful for veterinarians, veterinary students, laboratory and technical personnel, and farm managers.

The authors are highly knowledgeable and respected colleagues and should be congratulated for producing this valuable and updated addition to the poultry health literature.

Y. M. Saif

Professor and Head Emeritus
Diplomate ACVM, Charter Diplomate ACPV
Food Animal Health Research Program
OARDC/OSU
Wooster, OH 44691
USA

PREFACE

Infections with bacteria cause significant economic losses, mainly due to reduced weight gains or egg production, increased condemnations at slaughter and increased mortality. Furthermore, costs are caused by medication in case of disease as well by expenses for preventative measures like vaccination. Legislation and other regulations related to consumer protection and/or trade add to the administrative burden of poultry production.

Since bacteria play a significant role in poultry health and production, it is mandatory for everybody involved in growing poultry to know the basic characteristics of the most important bacterial poultry pathogens. The objective of this book is to present information on the most important bacterial diseases. Each chapter starts with a short introduction, followed by a description of the pathogen and an overview over transmission, pathogenesis and virulence factors. After that, we describe clinical signs and pathological lesions as well as laboratory methods for diagnosis and characterization of the bacterium. The chapters conclude with remarks on successful treatment and prevention by biosecurity or vaccination.

We have aimed to find a balance between concentrating on information that is directly relevant when dealing with the diseases and providing more scientific background information, which might help in the understanding of the disease and indicate developments that might become directly relevant in the future. For the same reason, we also refer to book chapters, review articles and original articles that will provide more detailed information on some aspects of the bacteria and the diseases mentioned in the text.

We hope that the reader will find this book both useful and interesting to read.

Hafez Mohamed Hafez and Rüdiger Hauck

TABLE OF CONTENTS

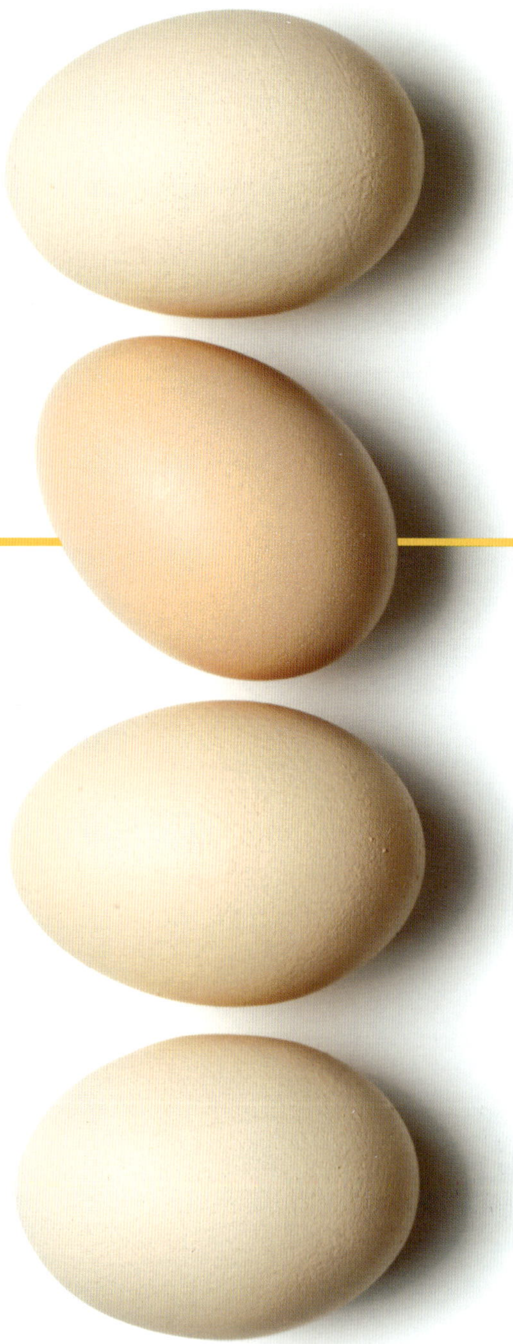

11 Botulism 95

12 Erysipelas 101

13 Infections with gram-positive cocci 107

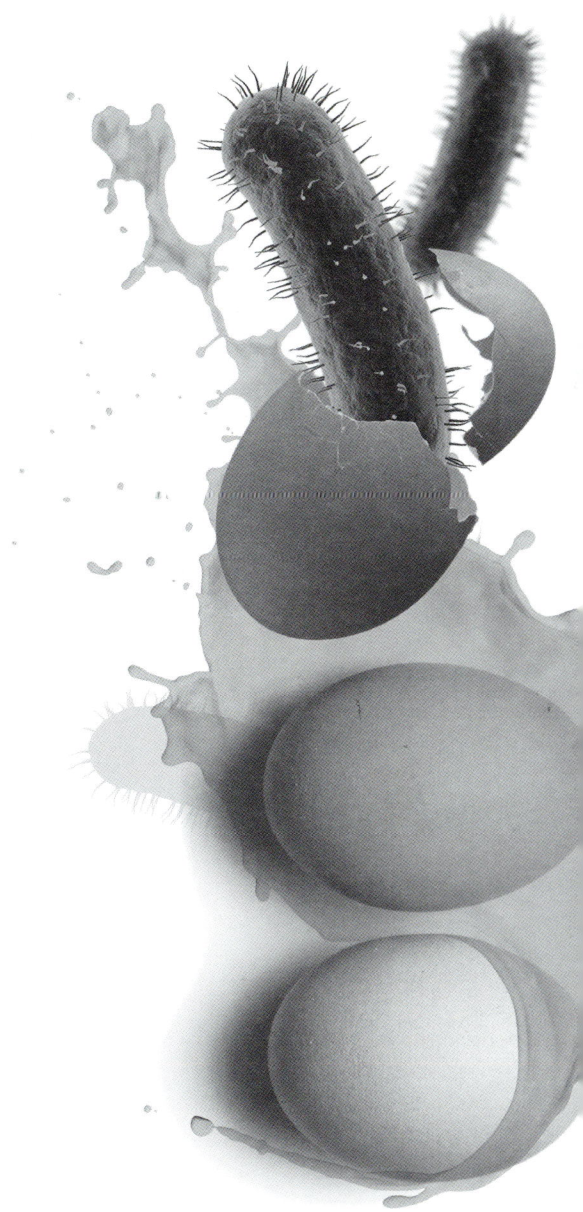

INTRODUCTION

Many bacteria are capable to infect poultry. Diseases caused by bacteria are responsible for significant economic losses, mainly due to increased mortality, reduced body weight gains or egg production and increased condemnation rate at slaughter. Furthermore, costs are caused by medication in case of disease as well by expenses for preventative measures like vaccination. Legislation and other regulations related to consumer protection and/or trade add to the administrative burden of poultry production.

Since bacteria play a significant role in poultry health and production, it is mandatory for everybody involved in this business to know the basic characteristics of the most important bacterial poultry pathogens. Knowing their basic characteristics like size, structure and metabolism, their ways and means of spreading, the pathogenesis of the diseases caused by them and the resulting clinical signs and pathological lesions helps to understand which methods of diagnosis are useful as well as which intervention strategies might work against the bacteria.

Basic characteristics of bacteria

Bacteria are larger than viruses and, as a consequence, they can be detected using a light microscope. Bacteria also have a larger genome than viruses. The genome of bacteria ranges between 160,000 and 12,200,000 base pairs and codes for a corresponding high number of different proteins. From the perspective of a diagnostician, these proteins are important because they constitute a high number of potential antigens, which may play a role in the detection of a bacterium or antibodies against it as well as in serotyping bacteria of one species. Furthermore, due to the high number of antigens, it is very difficult or even impossible to identify epitopes inducing neutralizing antibodies. Knowing such epitopes would be helpful for the design of vaccines.

Since many of the bacterial proteins are enzymes, they enable bacteria to have a complex metabolism of their own. Thus, most bacteria grow outside and without the presence of host cells, which makes isolation of these bacteria easier than isolation of viruses.

Table 1. Commonly used media and growth requirements for the bacteria covered in this book.

BACTERIA	COMMONLY USED MEDIA
Salmonella enterica	Grows on many media; for sensitive isolation, a three-stage procedure consisting of unspecific pre-enrichment in buffered peptone water, specific enrichment in liquid or semi-solid media at an increased temperature and selective agar is used.
Escherichia coli	Grows on many media; blood agar, MacConkey agar and Gassner agar are the most frequently used.
Thermophilic *Campylobacter* spp.	Fastidious; for selective enrichment, liquid medium like Preston-Bouillon or Bolton-Bouillon followed by charcoal containing selective agars like mCCDA or Karmali-Agar; also grows on blood agar; grows best at 42 °C and under microaerophilic conditions.
Pasteurella multocida	Dextrose starch agar, blood agar or trypticase soy agar.
Ornithobacterium rhinotracheale, *Riemerella anatipestifer*	Blood agar, might be supplemented with 0.5 µm/ml gentamicin and 0.5 µm/ml polymyxin to suppress growth of other bacteria; grows better under microaerophilic conditions.
Avibacterium paragallinarum	Fastidious; grows on blood agar in the presence of a V-factor producing nurse culture, often *Staphylococcus hyicus*; needs microaerophilic conditions.
Mycoplasma spp.	Very fastidious, slow growth; Frey's medium and PPLO broth are the most commonly used; both contain thallium and penicillin for selectivity.
Chlamydia psittaci	Isolation in various cell cultures or embryonated chicken eggs.
Clostridium perfringens, C. botulinum	Reinforced clostridial medium, blood agar, egg yolk agar; strictly anaerobe.
Erysipelothrix rhusiopathiae	Blood agar, MacConkey agar and triple sugar iron agar are the most commonly used.
Staphylococcus spp., *Streptococcus* spp.	Grow on many media; blood agar and MacConkey agar can be used.

On the other hand, the pathogenic bacteria are adapted to growing inside of hosts where many nutrients are readily available. The differences of the bacteria regarding their metabolism have to be taken into account when selecting suitable media for their isolation, but can also be used for identification of bacterial isolates. Table 1 lists and groups the bacteria presented in this book according to their growth requirements and suitable media for their isolation.

The structure and morphology of bacteria is another important criterion for identification of bacteria. The best-known classification scheme for bacteria is set according to their form and colour after Gram staining (Fig. 1). A plethora of other stains is used to visualize differences in the structure of the bacterial cell wall (Figs. 2 and 3).

In comparison to eukaryotic parasites, bacteria are less complex and smaller, and while many bacteria might infect a wide range of hosts, they do not have mandatory intermediate hosts as many parasites have. The lack of need for intermediate hosts facilitates the spread of bacteria, since it is not possible to just prevent contact between intermediate hosts and poultry to stop the infectious cycle. On the other hand, the less complicate life cycle of bacteria makes their *in vitro* culture easier.

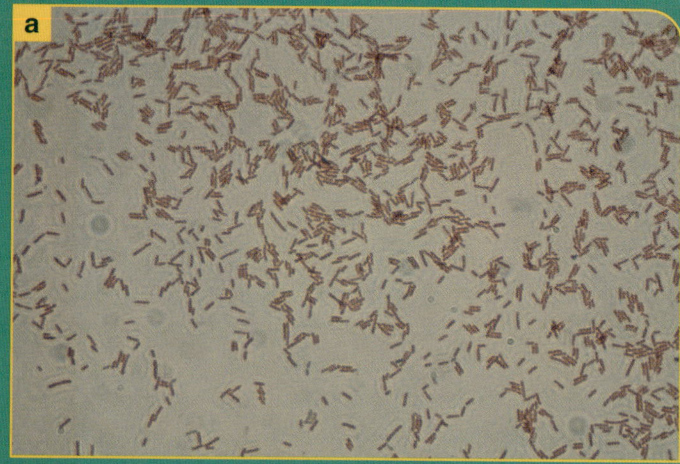

Figure 1. Various Gram-stained bacteria:
(a) Slender gram-negative rods (*Escherichia coli*).
(b) Pleomorphic gram-negative rods (*Ornithobacterium rhinotracheale*).
(c) Plump gram-positive rods (*Clostridium* sp.).
(d) Slender gram-positive rods (*Clostridium* sp.).
(e) Gram-positive cocci (*Enterococcus* sp.).

Poultry diseases caused by bacterial infections

Due to their connection to the environment and especially their function in exchanging metabolites with the environment, the respiratory tract and the gastrointestinal tract of poultry are most vulnerable and most often affected. The blood is the third important location where bacteria grow in the body and can cause diseases. The growth of bacteria in the blood is called septicaemia, while the mere presence of bacteria in the blood, without them multiplying, is called bacteraemia. Once the blood has transported bacteria throughout the body, bacteria can grow in virtually all organs and cause lesions there. An alternate way of bacteria to spread throughout the body is in the air sacs. Of the bacteria covered in this book, *Clostridium botulinum* is exceptional, since ingestions of *C. botulinum* toxins without infection with *C. botulinum* can cause disease.

Bacteria also differ significantly in the severity of the disease they cause. Some bacteria like *Pasteurella multocida*, *Salmonella* Gallinarum/*Salmonella* Pullorum or *Erysipelothrix rhusiopathiae* are the primary causative agents of severe diseases. Other bacteria like *Campylobacter* spp. and some *Salmonella* serovars are responsible for subclinical silent infections, but poultry products contaminated with them are of major public health concern. Still other bacterial species like *Ornithobacterium rhinotracheale*, *Mycoplasma* spp. or *Clostridium perfringens* cause only mild clinical signs and/or lesions on their own, but together with other pathogens and/or unfavourable environmental conditions they can lead to significant disease outbreaks. Many further bacteria fall somewhere between these above mentioned categories.

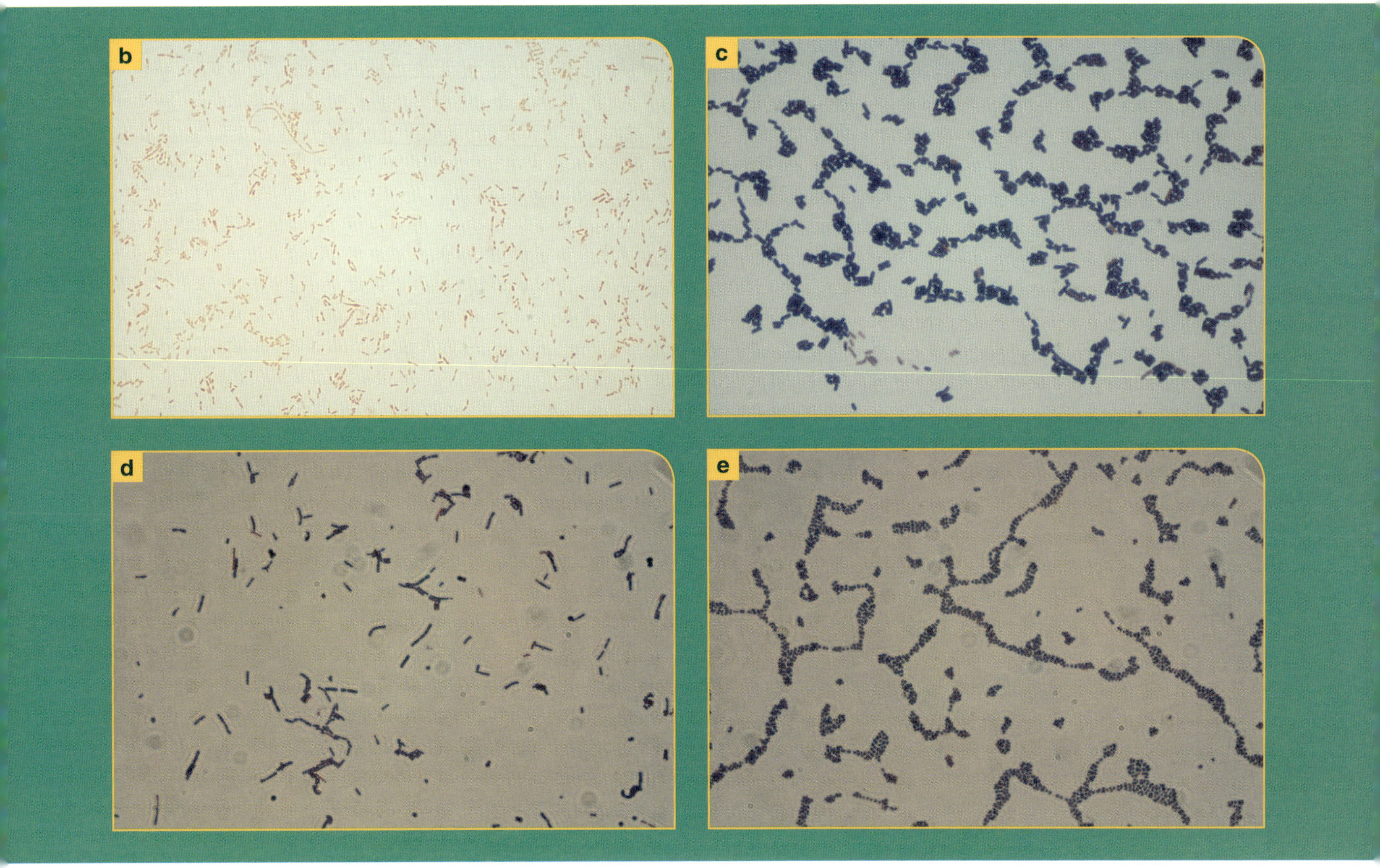

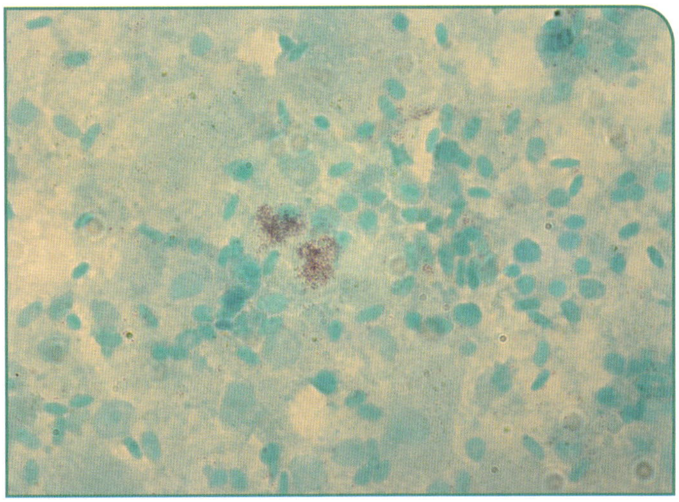

Figure 2. Chlamydial elementary bodies in an organ smear stained with Stamp stain.

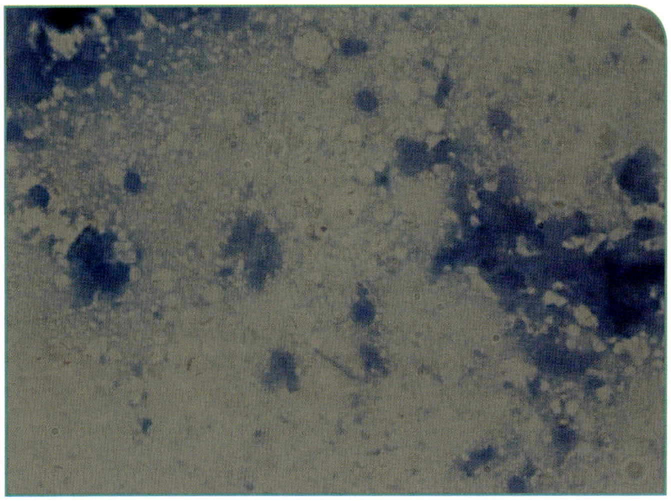

Figure 3. Acid-fast rods (*Mycobacteria*) in an organ smear stained with Ziehl-Neelsen stain.

Principals of diagnosis

Clinical signs and lesions caused by bacteria rarely allow a definite diagnosis, and thus confirmation in the laboratory is necessary.

For many bacteria, isolation followed by identification based on their morphology and metabolic profile is the method of choice to diagnose the disease.

However, isolation and identification, sometimes followed by typing, will take several days. Quicker and easier methods, which can be helpful with some diseases, are stained direct smears of organs with lesions or blood smears.

When isolation is tried, samples collection should be carried out using clean instruments, since conditions during transport of samples to the laboratory are critical. The transport should be done as fast as possible and samples should be shipped cooled in a media designed for that purpose. Transport media contain buffers for a stable pH and only a low amount of nutrients. They may also contain activated charcoal to neutralize toxins in the sample and inhibitors for microorganisms other than the suspected one. The aim is to keep the bacteria viable but to prevent overgrowth by other bacteria, which might be present in the sample.

If a transport under these conditions is not possible and/or for fastidious bacteria including obligate intracellular bacteria, detection of the bacterial genome by polymerase chain reaction (PCR) might be a preferable method. A properly validated PCR assay is sensitive, specific and fast. On the downside, not all bacteria can be typed without being isolated first. Furthermore, antibacterial sensitivity testing (AST) requires bacterial isolates.

Detection of antibodies is mostly used to test for absence of an infection or to monitor the success of vaccination. Detection of antibodies can be helpful in diagnosis if an increase in antibody titers is shown.

Today, enzyme-linked immunosorbent assay (ELISA) is the method of choice for antibody detection, since it gives fast and reliable results.

Furthermore, most ELISAs detect antibodies against all serotypes of a bacterial species. Other methods to detect antibodies include agar gel precipitation test (AGPT), serum agglutination and haemagglutination inhibition (HI) for some *Mycoplasma* strains, which tend to be more type-specific, but vary in their reliability and time and effort required.

Therapy of bacterial diseases

While bacteria have an active metabolism and a complex structure in common with eukaryotic cells, differences are large enough to allow some compounds to damage bacterial cells but not host cells. These drugs are called antibiotics or antimicrobials, with the latter expression also including antiparasitic agents. Almost all antibiotics are naturally occurring compounds or derivates of naturally occurring compounds. Microorganisms produce them as a means of defence against competing bacteria and, as a consequence, resistance mechanisms against antibiotics have co-evolved for a very long time. The massive production and use of antibiotics in the last 70 years made effective therapy of bacterial diseases possible, but has also caused a higher prevalence of antibacterial resistances. This renders some antibiotics almost useless in animals nowadays and might also pose a risk to human health.

In the interest of an effective therapy and to limit the spread of antibacterial resistance, antibiotics should be used only in a targeted way in order to minimize their useless administration.

Because therapy has to start as soon as possible, it is not feasible to wait for the result of AST, but AST of isolated bacteria keeps track of the resistance situation and will help in the selection of the right antibiotic in future cases. General concepts and detailed protocols for AST are published by the Clinical & Laboratory Standards Institute (CLSI) (CLSI, 2013). Knowledge of the spectrum of activity of antibiotics and pharmacological properties will also help in the selection of the right antibiotic (Table 2).

Following the instructions in the product information will also help to ensure that antibiotic therapy is effective.

Last, it is important to realize that for many bacteria, if not most, antibacterial therapy will mitigate clinical signs and lesions but not eliminate the pathogen from a flock. This applies e.g. for *Salmonella*, *Campylobactyer*, *Mycoplasma* or *E. coli*.

Prevention of bacterial diseases

The main ways to control any infectious disease are to prevent the introduction in an area supposed to be free from the infectious agent by biosecurity and regular monitoring. In case of the presence of infection in one area, measures should be taken to prevent the spread to other places. These measures might be enhanced by biosecurity,

Table 2. Most important antibacterial classes used to treat bacterial infections in poultry.

CLASS	IMPORTANT COMPOUNDS	MODE OF ACTION	SPECTRUM OF ACTIVITY	REMARKS
Aminoglycosides	Gentamicin, streptomycin, spectinomycin, neomycin	**Bactericidal**: inhibition of bacterial protein synthesis	Aerobic gram-negative bacteria	–
Aminopenicillins	Ampicillin, amoxicillin	**Bactericidal**: inhibition of bacterial cell walls synthesis	Broad spectrum	Cross-resistance with penicillins [1]
Beta-lactamase inhibitors	Clavulanic acid	Beta-lactamase inhibitor	Broad spectrum	Does not act against bacteria on its own; given in combination with amoxicillin
Diaminopyrimidines	Trimethoprim	**Bacteriostatic**: inhibits synthesis of folate	Aerobic bacteria	Usually given in combination with a sulfonamide ("potentiated sulfonamide")
Fluoroquinolones	Enrofloxacin	**Bactericidal**: inhibition of bacterial DNA replication	Broad spectrum	Easily induces resistances
Lincosamides	Lincomycin	**Bacteriostatic**: inhibition of bacterial protein synthesis	Gram-positive bacteria, mycoplasma	Cross-resistance with macrolides
Macrolides	Erythromycin, tilmicosin, tylosin	**Bacteriostatic**: inhibition of bacterial protein synthesis	Mainly gram-positive bacteria, mycoplasma, no Enterobacteriaceae	Cross-resistance with lincosamides and pleuromutilins [2]
Natural penicillins	Benzylpenicillin (penicillin G), penicillin V	**Bactericidal**: inhibition of bacterial cell walls synthesis	Gram-positive bacteria	Cross-resistance with aminopenicillins [1]
Pleuromutilins	Tiamulin	**Bacteriostatic**: inhibition of bacterial protein synthesis	Broad spectrum	Cross-resistance with macrolides; [2] toxicity in combination with ionophore antibiotics (coccidiostats)
Polypeptides	Colistin	**Bactericidal**: increases permeability of cell wall	Gram-negative bacteria	No absorption from the intestines; almost no resistances known
Sulfonamides	Sulfadimidin, sulfaclozin, sulfaquinoxalin	**Bacteriostatic**: inhibits synthesis of folate	Broad spectrum, including coccidia	Toxicity in combination with ionophore antibiotics (coccidiostats)
Tetracyclines	Tetracycline, oxytetracycline, chlortetracycline	**Bacteriostatic**: inhibition of bacterial protein synthesis	Broad spectrum	–

[1] Resistance against aminopenicillins indicates resistance against penicillins, but not vice versa.

[2] Resistance against pleuromutilins indicates resistance against macrolides, but not vice versa.

movement restriction, treatment, vaccination and, in some cases, eradication. Eradication policy and killing of flocks for disease control purposes are commonly applied in cases of suspicion or confirmed outbreaks with a considerable public health and/or economic impact.

Biosecurity and hygiene plans should be adopted for each farm. Farm owners, managers and workers should be involved in the design and implementation of the biosecurity plan. The aim is to create an environment where poultry are protected from carriers of infectious agents. Controlling the movement of people, animals, equipment, and vehicles in and out of the farm and within the farm area is essential.

Visitors are one of the major vectors and carriers of infectious agents. Visitors include supervisors, veterinarians, vaccination crews, catching crews, electricians, feed truck drivers, and other similar. Visitors can transmit diseases from one farm to another via dust on hands, hair, and clothing.

Good management, namely thorough cleaning and disinfection between flocks, water hygiene, adequate air quality and good litter will keep the infection pressure down and prevent clinical signs after infection. While these measures are essential, it is beyond the scope of this book to give detailed information on them.

Vaccination provides specific protection. For some bacteria, live attenuated vaccines, which induce a good local and cellular immune response, are available. Live vaccines are also suitable for the less laborious administration in the drinking water. For some vaccine strains, attenuation was achieved by adapting them to grow at a lower temperature than the body temperature of the host, so that they do not multiply efficiently in the host and are more easily dealt with by the immune system. Live bacterial vaccines can also be marker vaccines. Markers are a certain antibiotic resistance or auxotrophy, i.e. the inability to synthesize a required particular organic compound. Auxotrophic strains can have the added advantage of surviving for a shorter time in the environment.

Parenteral application of killed vaccines induces high antibody titers. They are especially effective when given as a booster vaccination. Due to the relative ease to culture bacteria, killed vaccines with bacterial antigens are comparatively inexpensive and the manufacture and use of autogenous vaccines is widespread.

As mentioned above, due to the diversity of antigens, it is very difficult to produce effective recombinant vaccines against bacteria.

Since the success of any disease control programme depends on the farm and personal sanitation, it is essential to incorporate education programmes about microorganisms, modes of transmission as well as awareness of the reasons behind such control programmes by people involved in poultry production.

References

CLSI. VET01-A4: Performance Standards for Antimicrobial Disk and Dilution Susceptibility Tests for Bacteria Isolated From Animals; Approved Standard - Fourth Edition; 2013.

BACTERIAL INFECTIONS

1 Salmonellosis

Overview

The genus *Salmonella* belongs to the family Enterobacteriaceae and all *Salmonella* covered in this book belong to the species *Salmonella enterica*. As all Enterobacteriaceae, *S. enterica* is a Gram-negative rod, cytochrome C oxidase negative and without the capability to form spores. Based on its antigens, *S. enterica* and its subspecies are divided in approximately 2700 serovars. The somatic (O) antigens, which are lipopolysaccharides by their chemical nature and heat stable, serve to define groups, which are designated by capital letters A through Z. Further groups are given numbers between 51 and 67. Serovars are further defined by their flagellar (H) antigens, which are proteins by their chemical nature and heat labile. Each antigenic variant is a serovar, which are systematically listed in the Kauffmann-White scheme (Grimont and Weill, 2007). To indicate that serovar names are not species names, the names of the serovars are capitalized, but not italicized.

Additionally, *Salmonella* can also be divided into three groups based on their host specificity and invasiveness (Hafez, 2001). Invasive *Salmonella* have the capability to "invade" the body from the intestinal lumen and thus infect organs, causing more serious disease. **Group 1** contains highly host-adapted and invasive serovars. Examples are *S.* Gallinarum in poultry or *S.* Typhi in humans. **Group 2** contains non-host-adapted and invasive serovars. *Salmonella* in this group are of most concern regarding public health, since some of them are capable to infect humans and food-producing animals and especially poultry can serve as reservoirs. There are approximately 10–20 serovars in this group. Currently, the most relevant serovars are *S.* Typhimurium, *S.* Enteritidis, *S.* Heidelberg, *S.* Hadar as well as *S.* Arizonae. **Group 3** contains non-host-adapted and non-invasive serovars, which are harmless for animals and humans. However, they are occasionally detected during monitoring for more important serovars. Most serovars of the genus *Salmonella* belong to this group. About 10 % of the known serovars have been detected in poultry. Motile *Salmonella* in poultry are called paratyphoid *Salmonella*.

Historically, *S.* Gallinarum and *S.* Pullorum were the most important *Salmonella* serovars in chickens. More recently, however, they have been almost completely eradicated from commercial poultry in industrialized countries and have only a low prevalence in backyard flocks. Thus, *S.* Gallinarum and *S.* Pullorum have lost relevance except in developing countries, while paratyphoid infections are regarded as more significant due to their zoonotic potential. *S.* Arizonae is a paratyphoid *Salmonella* and has some zoonotic potential, but its main importance as a causative agent is well documented for turkey flocks (Hafez, 2013).

Paratyphoid *Salmonella* infections

The importance of infections with paratyphoid *Salmonella* in poultry is twofold. First, contaminated eggs, poultry meat and meat products are regarded as one of the main sources of human *Salmonella*. When contaminated products are not adequately cooked, they will directly infect their consumers. Careless handling also poses a risk for cross-contamination of working surfaces and equipment in the kitchen, leading to cross-contamination of other foods. In recent years, significant improvements have been made in technology and hygienic practices at all stages of poultry production. As a consequence, the incidence of human salmonellosis has decreased in many countries, but the disease is still of concern and efforts to control it have to continue. The European Food Safety Authority (EFSA) has published several scientific opinions on a quantitative estimation of the public health impact of setting a new target for the reduction of *Salmonella* in laying hens, broilers as well as in turkeys (EFSA, 2010, 2011, 2012; summarized by Messens et al., 2013).

Chapter co-authored by Dr. H.L. Shivaprasad (California Animal Health and Food Safety Laboratory System, Tulare branch).

In addition to their relevance for public human health, salmonellosis and *Salmonella* infections can cause severe economic losses in poultry, which are caused by high mortality during the first 4 weeks of age, high medication costs, reductions in egg production in breeder flocks and poor chick quality.

Furthermore, there are high costs for eradication and control measures to protect birds and humans.

Aetiology

Paratyphoid *Salmonella* are non-host-adapted, and they can be invasive or non-invasive. In a certain region, some serovars may be predominant for a number of years before they disappear and one or several other serovars take their place. While decades ago *S.* Typhimurium was the most important reason of *Salmonella* food poisoning worldwide, since the early 1980s *S.* Enteritidis is regarded as at least as important. Recently, some notable outbreaks of salmonellosis in humans have been caused by *S.* Heidelberg in the USA, while in Europe, *S.* Hadar, *S.* Infantis and *S.* Virchow are regarded as problems.

In recent years, the number of cases of human salmonellosis in the European Union (EU) has steadily decreased. However, *Salmonella* is still the second most commonly reported gastrointestinal bacterial pathogen in humans after *Campylobacter*.

There was also a reduction of the prevalence of *S.* Enteritidis and *S.* Typhimurium in all types of commercial poultry and most member states met their reduction targets. Of all foodstuffs, fresh turkey meat had the highest proportion of *Salmonella*-positive samples, followed by broiler meat. Only 0.03 % of all table eggs were *Salmonella*-positive (EFSA, 2015).

Pathogenesis and transmission

The infection can be transmitted horizontally (laterally), mostly by the faecal-oral route, or vertically. *Salmonella* spread horizontally in feed, water, equipment and the general environment. They are fairly resistant and can survive or under favourable conditions even multiply outside their hosts. Virtually all vertebrates, including humans, rodents and pets as well as wild birds like waterfowl and pigeons. Rodents are regarded as a potential reservoir and responsible for spreading the infection from one house to another and for contaminating stored feed and raw materials. *Salmonella* have also been detected in different species of wild birds near poultry operations. They can enter not sufficiently secured houses or contaminate equipment of houses with their droppings. In addition, insects like the darkling beetle (*Alphitobius diaperinus*) are a potential source of *Salmonella* infection in chickens (Roche et al., 2009). Probably one of the most common sources for lateral spread of the organisms is the feed. Nearly every ingredient ever used in the manufacture of poultry feedstuffs has been shown at one time or another to contain *Salmonella*.

Vertical transmission happens through contaminated eggs laid by infected carriers, especially with *S.* Enteritidis. In between horizontal and vertical transmission lies early horizontal transmission. Early horizontal transmission happens in hatcheries, when contaminated and *Salmonella*-free eggs, either from the same or from different breeder flocks, are incubated together. Under these conditions, infection by aerosols containing *Salmonella* plays an important role and chicks are more susceptible to respiratory than to oral infection. Within a hatchery, *Salmonella* can spread via the ventilation, belt slots, door seals within hatchers and on all kinds of equipment. In consequence, the bacteria can continuously recycle from hatchers to hatched birds, from hatched birds to dust and equipment and back into the hatchers.

***Salmonella* spp. can persist for many years in a hatchery (Friend and Franson, 1999).**

After oral infection, *Salmonella* will replicate in the intestinal lumen and especially in the caeca. Virulent strains attach to the intestinal wall and invade host cells, most notably enterocytes and macrophages. Within the macrophages, in which they survive and grow in lysosomes, *Salmonella* are spread to other organs, most notably liver and spleen as well as to the ovaries. The ability to invade tissue in that way is probably the most important virulence determinant in young chicks. In older birds, invasion rarely happens (Turnbull and Snoeyenbos, 1974; Barrow et al., 1987).

Clinical signs

Clinical signs become apparent after 2 to 5 days. Mortality may be increased only very slightly, but can reach 20 % in young birds; in extreme cases, 80 % mortality and more have been reported. The outcome of an infection is dependent on the virulence of the causative serovar, infection pressure, age of birds, environmental conditions and presence of other, especially immunosuppressive infections. Clinical signs in young birds are non-specific and include weakness and somnolence, decreased food consumption, and ruffled feathers. Feathers, especially at the vent, are dirty with faeces as a consequence of diarrhoea. Infected birds huddle together near heat sources. Birds may die as a consequence of starvation and dehydration. Surviving birds will become emaciated and may be immunosuppressed (Gast, 2013).

Chickens older than 1 week usually show no or very little clinical signs even with systemic infections. The reasons for this age resistance are not well understood and remain under investigation.

Post mortem lesions

Common post mortem lesions are omphalitis and a persistent yolk sac (Figs. 1 and 2) as well as necrotic foci in liver (Fig. 3), spleen and heart muscle. Kidneys and spleen are frequently enlarged and congested (Fig. 4). In the intestine, a catarrhal and haemorrhagic enteritis may be present and the caecal lumen is frequently filled with a fibrinous, caseous core or with blood (Fig. 5). Hydropericardium,

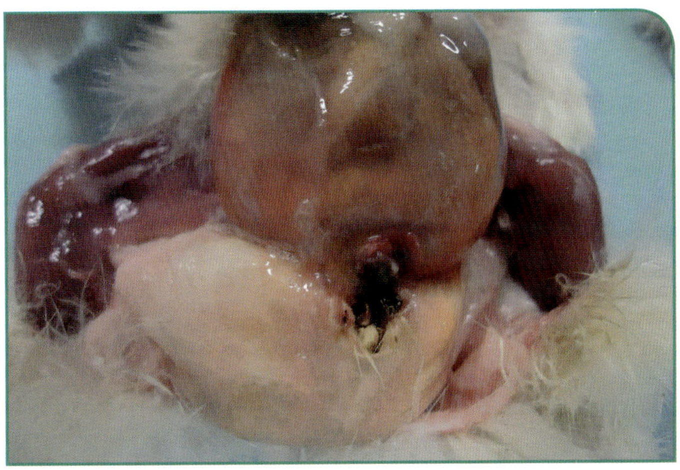

Figure 1. Omphalitis characterized by black crusts at the navel.

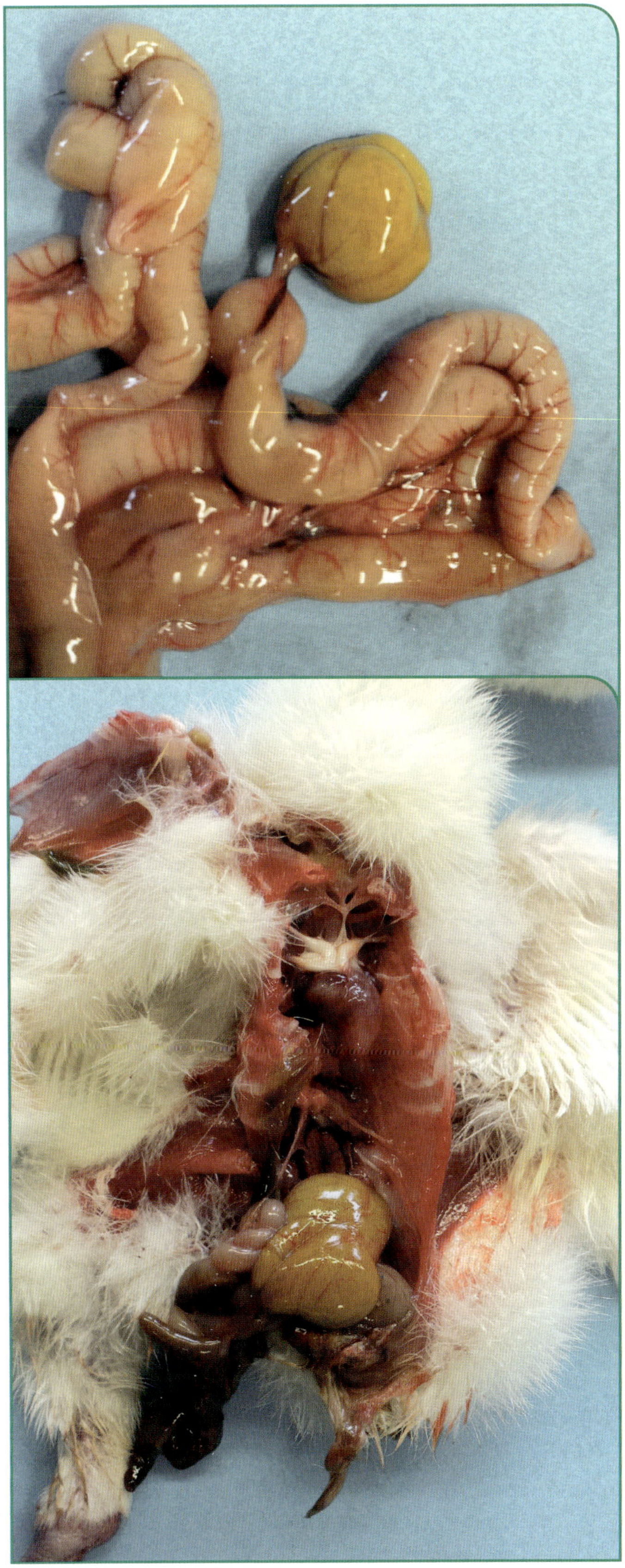

Figure 2. Persistent and inflamed yolk sac with greenish content.

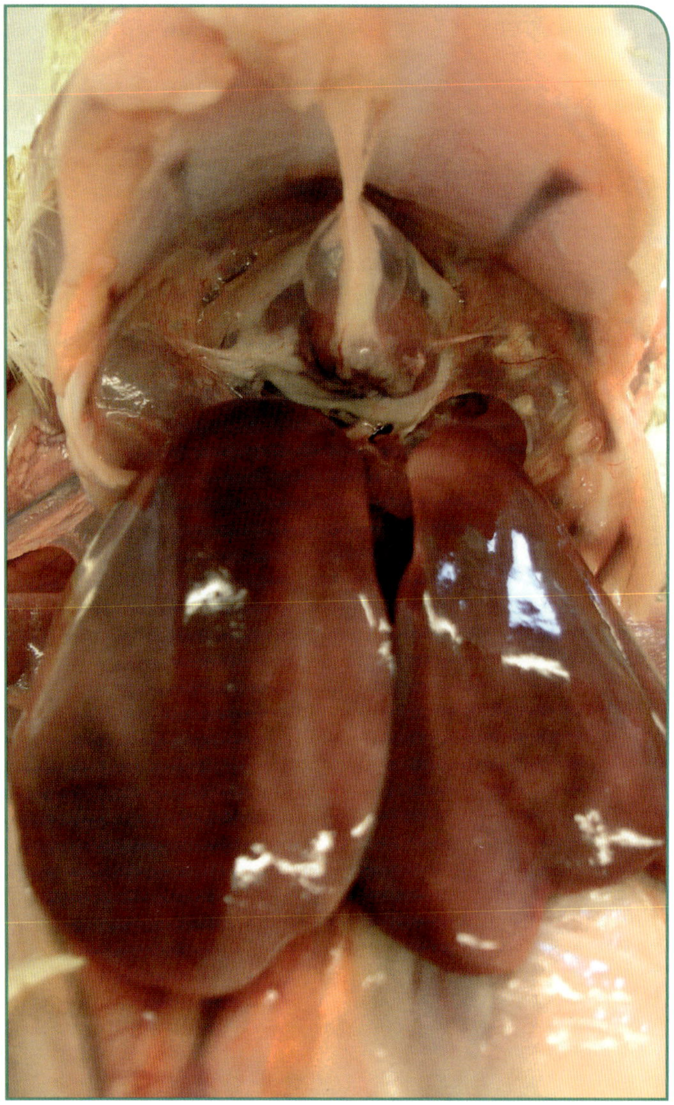

Figure 3. Liver with discoloured necrotic areas.

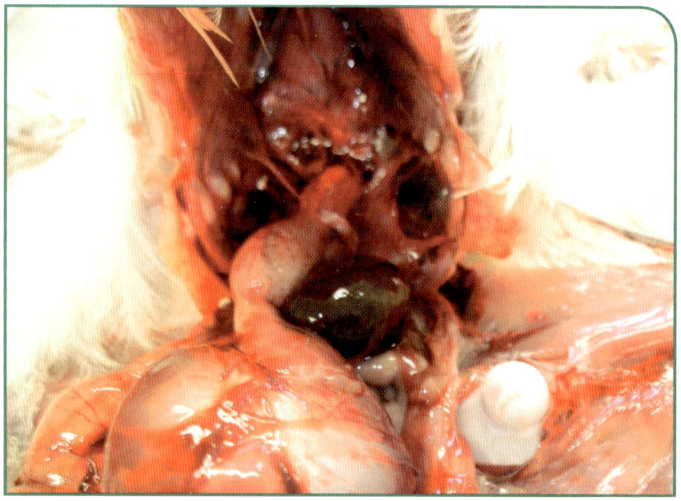

Figure 4. Enlarged and congested spleen with necrotic areas.

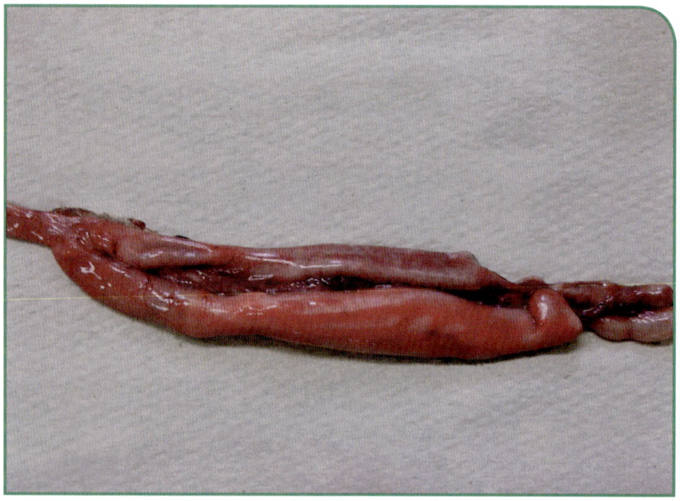

Figure 5. Caeca with fibrinous cores.

characterized by the presence of straw-coloured fluid in the heart sac or pericarditis, is another common finding (Fig. 6).

Diagnostic procedures

Clinical signs and lesions are of little value in diagnosis because, in many cases, the infection is not accompanied with clinical disease or lesions. Accurate diagnosis must be substantiated by isolation, identification of the causative bacteria and/or detection of antibodies using serological examination. In general, however, governmental regulation by diagnosis should be followed. Currently, in the EU the isolation of the organism is required by the legislation.

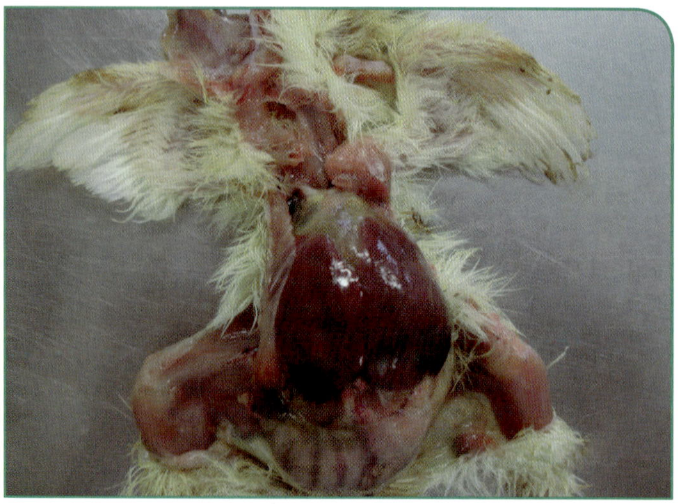

Figure 6. Hepatitis and pericarditis.

Detection of *Salmonella*, usually by isolation, is the most common method to confirm a presumptive diagnosis or to detect subclinical infections.

A large number of different samples can be used for isolation of *Salmonella*, depending on the circumstances. Suitable samples may be hatching eggs and dead-in-shell embryo or unabsorbed yolk sac to detect vertical transmission, heart blood, liver, spleen or kidney for systemic infections of chicks or older birds. To detect asymptomatic carriers, caecal content, faeces and environmental samples such as drag swabs, litter and dust can be taken.

The isolation procedure consists of culture in non-selective pre-enrichment and subsequent selective enrichment in liquid or semi-solid media, followed by transferring on selective agar. While the pre-enrichment will increase the number of organisms and revitalize stressed *Salmonella*, the selective enrichment will reduce gram-positive competing organisms. On the selective agar, *Salmonella* colonies can be recognized by a characteristic colour, depending on the agar used. Suspect colonies are confirmed by slide agglutination using poly- and monovalent sera. The exact procedure is laid down in ISO 6579 (Anon., 2002). Alternative molecular biological methods include detection after pre-enrichment by PCR and typing of isolates by microarray (Kim et al., 2006; Wattiau et al., 2008). For epidemiological purposes *Salmonella* isolates can be further typed by methods like macrorestriction analysis and pulsed-field gel electrophoresis (PFGE) or phage typing. The online database PulseNet offers a possibility to compare PFGE profiles of *Salmonella* isolates worldwide (Swaminathan et al., 2006).

Detection of antibodies in the serum by ELISA is possible. However, using this method it is not possible to determine which serovar is infecting the birds, since the detected antibodies are group specific. Antibody detection is not legally recognized for monitoring for food safety reasons.

Treatment

Antimicrobial drugs are highly effective in reducing mortality and clinical signs. However, treatment will not eliminate the infection. Since the treatment will also interfere with the detection of subclinically infected birds, the treatment of infected flocks not showing clinical signs with the intention to get a *Salmonella*-free flock is forbidden in the EU. In some cases, for example in the interest of animal welfare, the use of antimicrobials can be permitted (EC, 2006).

Control

The emphasis of any *Salmonella* control programme has to be to prevent the introduction of the bacteria into a flock. The main routes of entry for *Salmonella* are vertically infected chicks as discussed above, feed, fomites and other animals, including rodents.

In order to minimize the risk of vertical transmission, the production pyramid has to be cleaned from the top by applying rigorous biosecurity measures in primary breeders, grandparent and parent flocks and by close monitoring of these flocks.

Hatching egg sanitation will help reduce the rate of vertical transmission, in case the infection of the dams is missed. Pelletized feed should be free of *Salmonella*, since the bacteria will not survive the heat and pressure. However, great care has to be taken at the feed mill to avoid recontamination after pelletizing by strict separation of the ingredients, which might be contaminated with *Salmonella*, and the finished feed. Non-pelleted feed should be tested for *Salmonella* contaminations. Surface water might be contaminated with *Salmonella* and should be treated.

To prevent introduction of *Salmonella* into a flock by fomites and animals, the normal biosecurity measures, including cleaning and disinfection of any equipment entering the poultry house and rodent control, have to be vigorously applied.

The success of any biosecurity protocol depends on the compliance of the personnel. Thus, it is essential to raise awareness and to educate everybody involved in poultry production about microorganisms and their modes of transmission. In Europe, the EU has decreed targets for the reduction of the prevalence of *Salmonella* in poultry flocks (EC, 2003). Hafez (2010) summarized the control approaches of *Salmonella* infections in poultry in the EU.

In case a flock is infected with *Salmonella*, the use of competitive exclusion products as well as various pre- and probiotics will help to decrease duration and extent of shedding of *Salmonella*. This will decrease the risk for consumers. Products from these flocks should not be sold untreated to customers. Inactivated and live vaccines are commercially available against *S.* Typhimurium and *S.* Enteritidis. Their use, too, will decrease the shedding of *Salmonella*. Live vaccines are either resistant against certain antibiotics or auxotroph i.e. their growth is dependent on certain compounds, which field strains do not require. These markers make it possible to differentiate vaccine strains from field strains in the case of re-isolation during monitoring.

After an infection with *Salmonella*, the whole premises and all equipment have to be thoroughly cleaned and disinfected. While commonly used disinfectants are theoretically effective against *Salmonella*, in practice effective disinfection is difficult. Organic matter will reduce the activity of the disinfectants; furthermore, cleaning and disinfection must reach all possible spots like cracks in the wall or the roof construction where *Salmonella* might remain and be a source of infection for the next flock. *Salmonella* can stay infective in dust for months (Davies and Wray, 1994). They can also survive in biofilms in water pipes, which have to be cleaned and disinfected thoroughly between flocks (Schonewille et al., 2012).

Since December 2010, fresh poultry meat may not be placed on the market for consumers when *Salmonella* was detected in a flock. Instead the meat must be treated by heat or otherwise to eliminate *Salmonella* before being sold to consumers (EC, 2003). Furthermore, *Salmonella*-positive flocks should be slaughtered after *Salmonella*-negative flocks to avoid cross-contamination at the processing plant.

The last protective measures against human salmonellosis have to be taken by the consumers themselves, so raising awareness in a matter-of-fact way and education about how to handle raw animal products and especially poultry products are necessary.

Salmonella Arizonae infections

S. Arizonae falls under the definition of paratyphoid *Salmonella*. However, there are differences which set *S.* Arizonae apart from the other paratyphoid *Salmonella*. Arizonosis, the infection due to *S.* Arizona, can cause high mortality and reduced production in infected turkey flocks and reduce the hatchability. It is a serious problem in the turkey industry (Crespo et al., 2004). There are only few reports about the infection of chickens with *S.* Arizonae (Silva and Hipolito, 1978).

Aetiology

In contrast to the previously discussed *Salmonella*, *S.* Arizonae is not a member of the subspecies *S. enterica* ssp. *enterica*, but constitutes a subspecies of its own, *S. enterica* ssp. *arizonae*. *S. enterica* ssp. *enterica* and *S. enterica* ssp. *arizonae* differ in various biochemical tests, including β-galactosidase (OPNG) and gelatinase test. Currently, 99 *Salmonella* serovars are members of this subspecies (Grimont and Weill, 2007).

While warm-blooded animals are regarded as the usual habitat of *S. enterica* ssp. *enterica*, cold-blooded animals, especially reptiles, and environment are the usual habitat of *S. enterica* ssp. *arizonae* (Grimont and Weill, 2007).

However, the host range of *S.* Arizonae is very wide, and there are reports of human infections. Usually, reptiles are the source of these infections.

Pathogenesis and transmission

In most cases, birds acquire the infection vertically from breeder flocks; horizontal transmission seems to be less important in comparison (Crespo et al., 2004).

Clinical signs

Clinical signs of arizonosis in turkeys are identical to those in diseases caused by other *Salmonella* species. Affected poults show general depression and pasty vent due to diarrhoea as described above. In addition, uni- or bilateral blindness due to inflammation of the eyes, central nervous symptoms like uncoordinated movements, convulsions, twisted neck and torticollis can occur (Fig. 7). The latter signs might be either consequences of infections of the

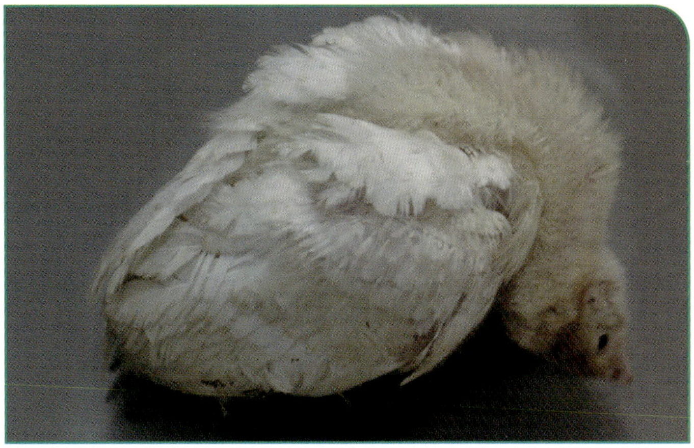

Figure 7. Turkey poult with neurological signs due to encephalitis caused by *Salmonella* Arizonae. Image courtesy of Dr. H.L. Shivaprasad (California Animal Health and Food Safety Laboratory System, Tulare branch).

brain or the inner ear (Shivaprasad et al., 2006). The signs of infection can be suppressed by antibiotic treatment of poults at the hatchery. Mortality can vary widely between 1 % and 50 %. Morbidity and mortality are highly dependent on the age. Most of the outbreaks occur in turkeys younger than 3 weeks of age, but increased mortality can continue after an outbreak through 5 weeks after hatch. Surviving birds will be runted and the flock will be uneven in size (Shivaprasad, 2013).

Older turkeys can become infected, but usually do not develop clinical signs apart from decreased egg production and fertility of breeder flocks. Hatchability of eggs from breeder flocks infected with *S.* Arizonae can also be decreased.

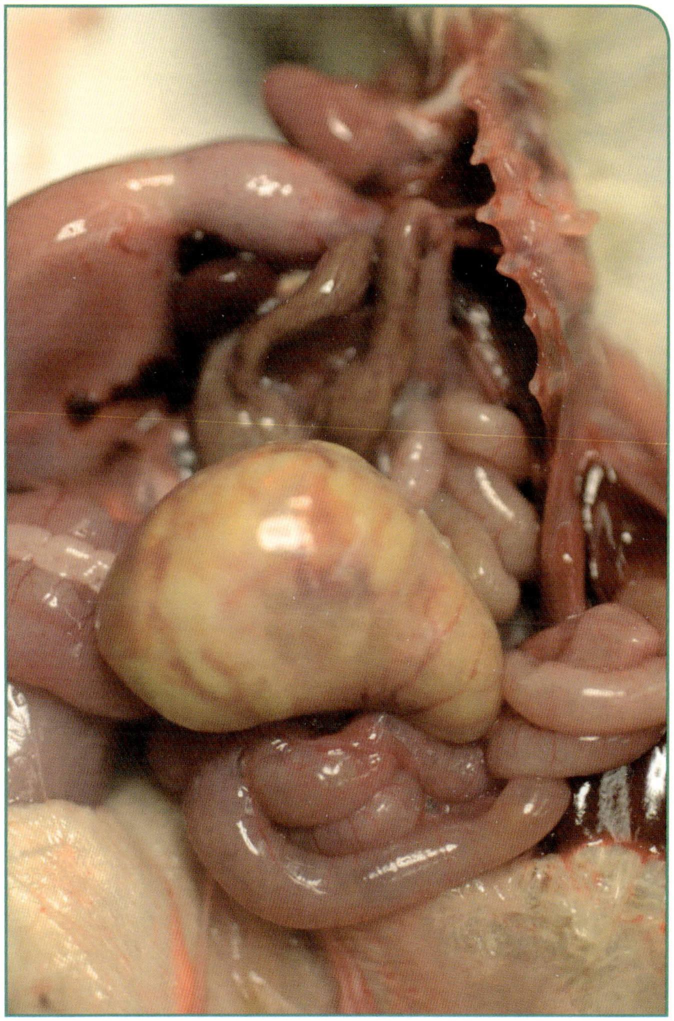

Figure 8. Yolk sac infection in a turkey poult due to *Salmonella* Arizonae. Image courtesy of Dr. H.L. Shivaprasad (California Animal Health and Food Safety Laboratory System, Tulare branch).

Post mortem lesions

Lesions at post mortem resemble closely those described for other paratyphoid *Salmonella*. Yolk sac infections (Fig. 8) and the accumulation of fibrinous exudate in caecal lumens (Fig. 9), body cavity and air sacs, brain and inner ear as well as especially in the eye seem to be more frequent. Distended gallbladder with ulcers is another lesion indicative for *S.* Arizonae, but also for other infections with other *Salmonella* (Shivaprasad, 2013).

The same principles for laboratory diagnosis, treatment and control outlined above for other paratyphoid *Salmonella* are applied to *S.* Arizonae. There are no vaccines against *S.* Arizonae (Hafez, 2013).

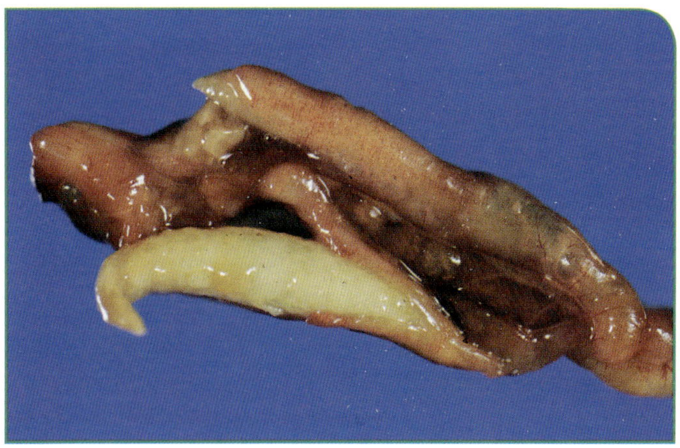

Figure 9. Typhlitis in a turkey poult due to *Salmonella* Arizonae. Image courtesy of Dr. H.L. Shivaprasad (California Animal Health and Food Safety Laboratory System, Tulare branch).

Salmonella Gallinarum infections (fowl typhoid) and *Salmonella* Pullorum infections (pullorum disease)

Fowl typhoid and pullorum disease are septicaemic infections caused by *S.* Gallinarum and *S.* Pullorum, respectively. Fowl typhoid affects primarily older chickens and turkeys, even though outbreaks with significant morbidity and mortality in younger birds have been described and experimentally reproduced. Pullorum disease mostly affects birds younger than 3 weeks. Outbreaks in older chickens and turkeys are rare.

Aetiology

Due to the differences between the disease they cause as well as between their biochemical and molecular biological properties, *S.* Gallinarum and *S.* Pullorum have been regarded as two different serovars for a long time. Currently, *S.* Pullorum is classified as a biovar of *S.* Gallinarum (Grimont and Weill, 2007). Sometimes the serovar is referred to *S.* Gallinarum-Pullorum (Shivaprasad and Barrow, 2013). In the following, the name *S.* Gallinarum will be used for simplicity, while indicating differences between the two diseases where necessary.

Based on its somatic O-antigen, *S.* Gallinarum belongs to group D. It is unique in that it lacks H-antigens and thus is non-motile.

Pathogenesis and transmission

In principle, *S.* Gallinarum is spread in the same way as described for paratyphoid *Salmonella* above, i.e. horizontally as well as vertically. Feed plays only a minor role as source of infection, while vertical transmission is relatively more important than for paratyphoid *Salmonella*.

It is noteworthy that even though *S.* Gallinarum is classified as host specific, it can in fact infect not only chickens, turkeys and other gallinaceous birds, but also ducks, sparrows, parrots, ostriches and even a wide range of mammals including humans (Shivaprasad and Barrow, 2013). These animals may act as living vectors, but very rarely develop disease after infection. The pathogenesis is similar as outlined above for paratyphoid *Salmonella*.

Clinical signs

First clinical signs become visible after 3 to 5 days after horizontal infection. In the case of vertical infections, the number of dead-in-shell embryos is increased; sometimes clinical signs become apparent only 4 or 5 days after hatch. The course of the disease can extend over 2 to 3 weeks and reoccur intermittently.

The signs of both diseases are similar, not characteristic and may include all organ systems. They include somnolence and listlessness, increased thirst as well as anorexia. Diseased chicks and poults have whitish diarrhoea, which is visible at the vent feathers ("pasty vent"). In older birds, diarrhoea is usually greenish-yellow. Respiratory distress due to pneumonia can also occur. Other symptoms that are sometimes present include conjunctivitis, swelling of joints and synovial sheaths (Fig. 10) with resulting lameness as well as nervous symptoms in rare cases. When infected birds are in lay, egg production, fertility and hatchability will be decreased and may be the only signs.

Diseased birds might withdraw from healthy birds to the walls of the house. The body temperature may increase before birds die. Some birds may die suddenly without previous clinical signs. Surviving birds will be poorly feathered and will show retarded growth; the flock will be uneven in size. After infections, birds will frequently remain carriers spreading the bacteria for a long time.

As the severity of the clinical signs, mortality is highly variable between 10 % and close to 100 % over the course of the disease. The outcome of infection is mostly depending on the virulence of the causative strain and on the age at infection.

Other factors influencing morbidity and mortality are the genetic background of the birds, infection pressure and management.

Post mortem lesions

In peracute cases, post mortem lesions may be absent in young chicks and poults. After a more protracted course of the disease, lesions can be seen in all organs. They include injected subcutaneous blood vessels, congested and dark skeletal muscles that may also appear as if partially cooked. Liver, heart, spleen and kidneys are enlarged and may have necrotic spots (Fig. 11); the liver can also have a bronze-like colour and be friable. Histopathological lesions vary, including congestion, infiltration of inflammatory cells and accumulation of fibrin. Necrotic foci and nodules are visible in myocardium, liver, pancreas or gizzard. The lungs are congested with small grey areas of focal necrosis.

Lesions in the intestines are more variable. A caseous, sometimes bloody core in the caeca is considered typical for pullorum disease. Histopathology will show extensive necrosis of the mucosa and submucosa. In contrast, fowl typhoid more often causes haemorrhagic enteritis and, in turkeys, ulcers in the duodenum. The content can also be more mucoid. The intestinal wall may be thickened in young birds or more flaccid in older birds. Many chicks and poults have persistent yolk sacs, with little or no signs of inflammation, but the yolk may be creamy or pasty (Fig. 12).

In adult birds, inflammation of the reproductive tract may be the only lesion. In male birds, the testes may be atrophied with thickening of tunica albuginea and multiple abscesses. In hens, the ovary follicles are discoloured with

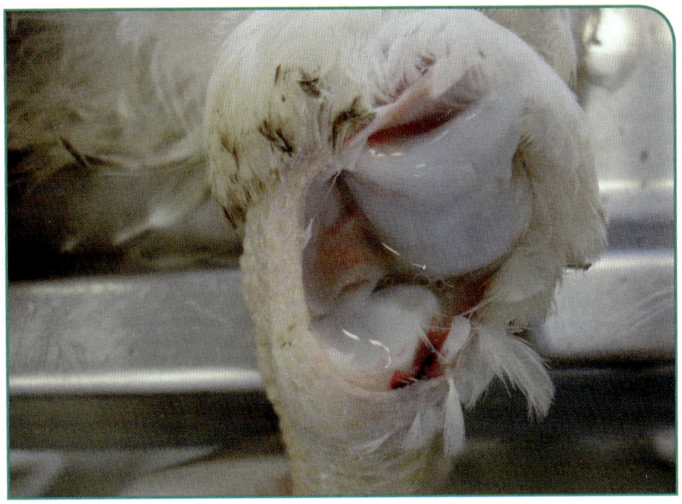

Figure 10. Inflamed hock joint filled with clear excess fluid

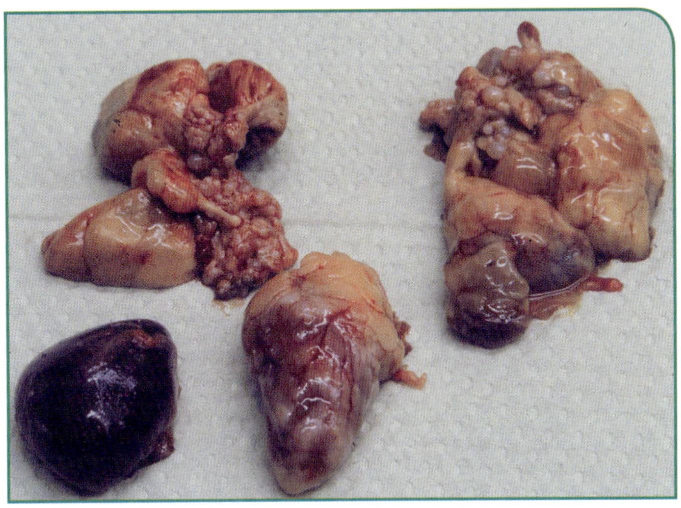

Figure 11. Enlarged and inflamed liver and heart with necrotic areas.

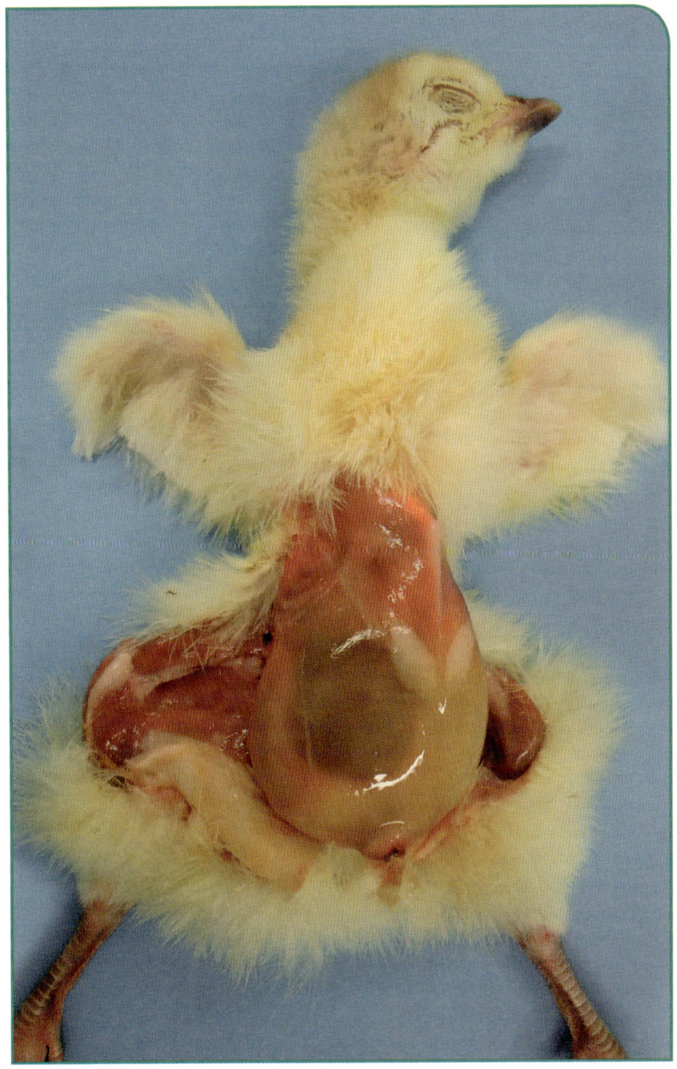

Figure 12. 1–day-old chick with inflamed yolk sac due to infection with *Salmonella* Pullorum.

a thickened capsule and oily or caseous content. They may also be pedunculated. The ovary may be haemorrhagic (Figs. 13 and 14). Microscopically, infiltration of heterophils, fibrin and bacterial colonies are visible in the coagulated yolk, surrounded by multinucleated giant cells more inflammatory cells. Often, the lumen of the oviduct contains caseous exudate. The lesions of ovary and oviduct may cause abdominal ovulation leading to extensive peritonitis.

Even without lesions in the reproductive tract, polyserositis is a common feature in older birds.

Diagnostic procedures

Presumptive diagnosis based on clinical signs and gross lesions has to be confirmed by isolation of *S.* Gallinarum from any of the affected organs. *S.* Gallinarum will grow on the most commonly used media like blood agar or MacConkey agar, and direct culture can be tried. The use of selective media like selenite cystine broth, tetrathionate broth or Rappaport–Vassiliadis broth may be helpful to prevent contamination with other bacteria in the case of intestinal samples or decomposed samples (Anon., 2012). It should be noted that the use of semisolid selective media for isolation of paratyphoid *Salmonella* will yield false-negative results, since *S.* Gallinarum lacks flagella and thus is immobile. Suspect colonies can be identified by slide agglutination test.

Historically, the detection of antibodies by various methods was and is used for monitoring purposes. Rapid agglutination tests using stained antigen are the most commonly used tests. In the field, whole blood can be investigated; in the laboratory, serum is the preferred sample. Since the disease is regarded as eradicated in industrialized countries, recently no commercially available antigen for this test was available in the EU. Cross-reactions with antibodies against group D *Salmonella*, other *Salmonella* and even other bacteria are frequent.

Commercially available ELISAs to detect antibodies against *S.* Enteritidis will also detect antibodies against *S.* Gallinarum and other group D *Salmonella*.

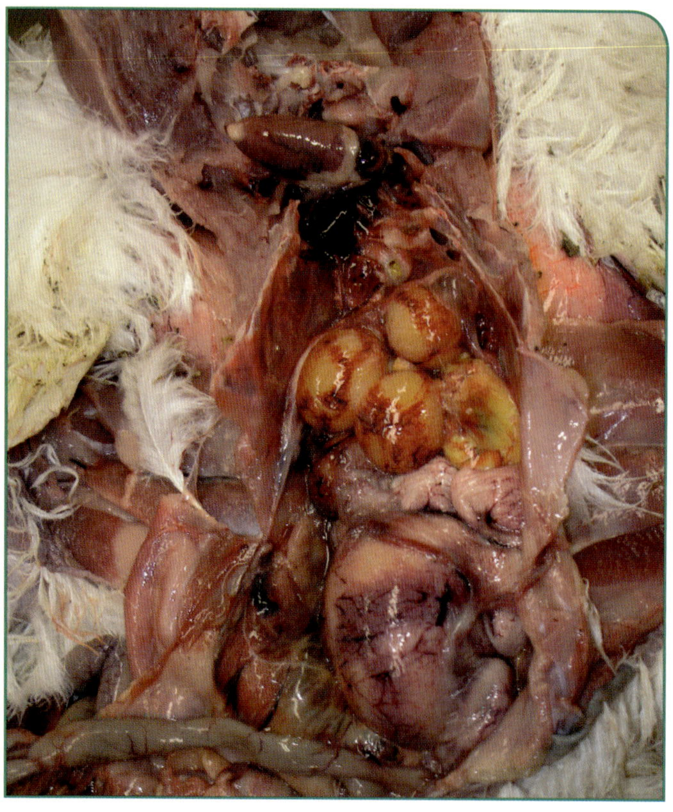

Figure 13. Inflamed ovary with haemorrhagic follicles.

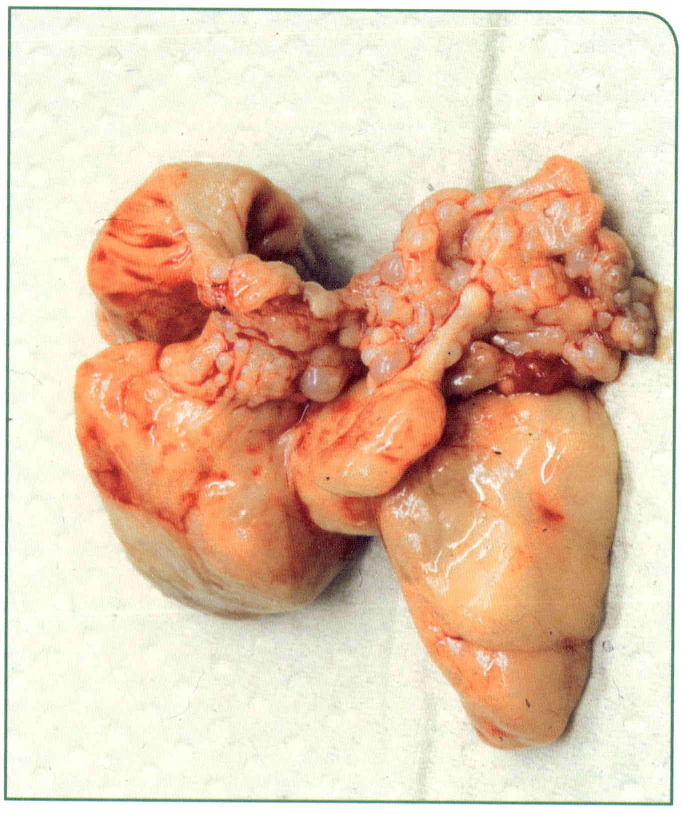

Figure 14. Severely inflamed ovary; follicles are discoloured with a thickened capsule and oily or caseous content.

Treatment

As with paratyphoid *Salmonella*, treatment with sulfonamides, tetracyclines or aminoglycosides will reduce mortality and clinical signs. However, since it will not clear the infection, treatment will create carriers. It should therefore be avoided and infected birds should be culled.

Control

Control of *S.* Gallinarum is similar to the principles for control of paratyphoid *Salmonella*.

Since *S.* Gallinarum is less resistant in the environment than paratyphoid *Salmonella* and less likely to have reservoirs in wild animals, elimination of carriers in pedigree, grandparent and breeder flocks has resulted in the near complete eradication from commercial poultry.

This was achieved by large scale monitoring programmes involving considerable efforts.

In some countries, live or inactivated vaccines are available and are in use. The downside of their use is that they interfere with monitoring and that the achieved immunity is sufficient to prevent disease but not infection, thus possibly creating reservoirs that are difficult to detect.

In many countries, fowl typhoid and pullorum disease are reportable diseases, and both diseases are listed as notifiable by the OIE.

References

Anon. Chapter 2.3.11 - Pullorum disease and fowl typhoid. In: OIE Terrestrial Manual. 2012; http://www.oie.int/fileadmin/Home/eng/Health_standards/tahm/2.03.11_FOWL_TYPHOID.pdf

Anon. ISO 6579:2002 - Microbiology of food and animal feeding stuffs - Horizontal method for the detection of Salmonella spp.

Barrow PA, Huggins MB, Lovell MA and Simpson JM. Observations on the pathogenesis of experimental Salmonella typhimurium infection in chickens. *Research in Veterinary Science*. 1987; 42: 194–199.

Crespo R, Jeffrey JS, Chin RP, Sentíes-Cué G and Shivaprasad HL. Phenotypic and Genotypic Characterization of Salmonella arizonae from an Integrated Turkey Operation. *Avian Diseases*. 2004; 48: 344–350.

Davies RH and Wray C. Salmonella pollution in poultry units and associated enterprises. In: Pollution in Livestock Production Systems, edited by I Dewi, H Ohmed and IFM Marai, eds. CABI Publishing Wallingford, Oxon, UK. 1994; pp. 137–165.

EC. Regulation (EC) No 2160/2003 of the European Parliament and of the Council of 17 November 2003 on the control of salmonella and other specified foodborne pathogens. *Official Journal of the European Union*. 2003; L 325: 1–15.

EC. Regulation (EC) No 1177/2006 of 1 August 2006 implementing Regulation (EC) No 2160/2003 of the European Parliament and of the Council as regards requirements for the use of specific control methods in the framework of the national programmes for the control of salmonella in poultry. *Official Journal of the European Union*. 2006; L 212: 3–5.

EFSA. Scientific Opinion on a quantitative estimation of the public health impact of setting a new target for the reduction of Salmonella in laying hens. *EFSA Journal*. 2010; 8: 1546.

EFSA. Scientific Opinion on a quantitative estimation of the public health impact of setting a new target for the reduction of Salmonella in broilers. *EFSA Journal*. 2011; 9: 2106.

EFSA. Scientific Opinion on an estimation of the public health impact of setting a new target for the reduction of Salmonella in turkeys. *EFSA Journal*. 2012; 10: 2616.

EFSA. The European Union summary report on trends and sources of zoonoses, zoonotic agents and food-borne outbreaks in 2013. *EFSA Journal*. 2015; 13: 3991.

Friend M and Franson JC. Salmonellosis. In: Field manual of wildlife diseases – general field procedures and diseases of birds, eds. USGS. 1999; pp. 99–109.

Gast RK. Paratyphoid infections. In: Diseases of Poultry, edited by DE Swayne, JR Glisson, LR McDougald, LK Nolan, DL Suarez and V Nair, eds. Wiley-Blackwell Ames, Iowa, USA. 2013; pp. 693–706.

Grimont PAD and Weill F-X. Antigenic formulae of the Salmonella serovars. 9th edition. 2007; https://www.pasteur.fr/sites/www.pasteur.fr/files/wklm_en.pdf

Hafez HM. Salmonella infections in poultry: diagnosis and control. *Periodicum Biologorum*. 2001; 103: 103–113.

Hafez HM. Salmonella infections in poultry: Control approaches in the European Union. *Turkiye Klinikleri Journal of Veterinary Science*. 2010; 1(2): 80–88

Hafez HM. Salmonella infections in turkeys. In: Salmonella in Domestic Animals, edited by PA Barrow and U Methner, eds. CABI Publishing, ISBN 13: 978 1 84593902 1. 2013; pp. 193–220.

Kim S, Frye JG, Hu J, Fedorka-Cray PJ, Gautom R and Boyle DS. Multiplex PCR-Based Method for Identification of Common Clinical Serotypes of Salmonella enterica subsp. enterica. *Journal of Clinical Microbiology*. 2006; 44: 3608–3615.

Messens W, Vivas-Alegre L, Bashir S, Amore G, Romero-Barrios P and Hugas M. Estimating the Public Health Impact of Setting Targets at the European Level for the Reduction of Zoonotic Salmonella in Certain Poultry Populations. *International Journal of Environmental Research and Public Health*. 2013; 10: 4836–4850.

Roche AJ, Cox NA, Richardson LJ, Buhr RJ, Cason JA, Fairchild BD and Hinkle NC. Transmission of Salmonella to broilers by contaminated larval and adult lesser mealworms, Alphitobius diaperinus (Coleoptera: Tenebrionidae). *Poultry Science*. 2009; 88: 44–48.

SCHONEWILLE E, NESSE LL, HAUCK R, WINDHORST D, HAFEZ HM AND VESTBY LK. Biofilm building capacity of Salmonella enterica strains from the poultry farm environment. *FEMS Immunology and Medical Microbiology*. 2012; 65: 360–365.

SHIVAPRASAD HL. Arizonosis. In: Diseases of Poultry, edited by DE Swayne, JR Glisson, LR McDougald, LK Nolan, DL Suarez and V Nair, eds. Wiley-Blackwell Ames, Iowa, USA. 2013; pp. 706–713.

SHIVAPRASAD HL AND BARROW PA. Pullorum disease and fowl typhoid. In: Diseases of Poultry, edited by DE Swayne, JR Glisson, LR McDougald, LK Nolan, DL Suarez and V Nair, eds. Wiley-Blackwell Ames, Iowa, USA. 2013; pp. 678–693.

SHIVAPRASAD HL, CORTES P AND CRESPO R. Otitis interna (labyrinthitis) associated with Salmonella enterica arizonae in turkey poults. *Avian Diseases*. 2006; 50: 135–138.

SILVA EN AND HIPOLITO O. Salmonella strains isolated from the digestive tract of breeding chickens and apparently normal turkeys and in chick embryos. *Proc. World's Poultry Congress*. 1978; 16: 701–706.

SWAMINATHAN B, GERNER-SMIDT P, NG L-K, LUKINMAA S, KAM K-M, ROLANDO S, GUTIÉRREZ EP AND BINSZTEIN N. Building PulseNet International: an interconnected system of laboratory networks to facilitate timely public health recognition and response to foodborne disease outbreaks and emerging foodborne diseases. *Foodborne Pathogens and Disease*. 2006; 3: 36–50.

TURNBULL PC AND SNOEYENBOS GH. Experimental salmonellosis in the chicken. 1. Fate and host response in alimentary canal, liver, and spleen. *Avian Diseases*. 1974; 18: 153–177.

WATTIAU P, WEIJERS T, ANDREOLI P, SCHLIKER C, VEKEN HV, MAAS HME, VERBRUGGEN AJ, HECK MEOC, WANNET WJ, IMBERECHTS H AND VOS P. Evaluation of the Premi Test Salmonella, a commercial low-density DNA microarray system intended for routine identification and typing of Salmonella enterica. *International Journal of Food Microbiology*. 2008; 123: 293–298.

2 Colibacillosis

Infection with *Escherichia coli* is the most common and economically significant cause of increased morbidity and mortality leading to immense economical losses. *E. coli* is part of the natural bacterial flora of the intestines of chickens and many other birds and mammals. Consequently, *E. coli* is nearly ubiquitous. The bacterium can act as a primary and/or secondary pathogen and a lot of research effort has gone into determining virulence factors and classifying *E. coli* isolates based on their presence. Isolates capable to act as primary pathogens are designated as Avian Pathogenic *E. coli* (APEC).

E. coli can cause or be involved in various distinct disease conditions, which can be systemic or localized. The most important systematic infection is colisepticaemia. In the course of the septicaemia, the bacteria can infect virtually all organs. In addition, coligranulomatosis (Hjärre's disease) is also considered a systemic infection. Localized infections include omphalitis and yolk sac inflammation, swollen head syndrome (SHS), coliform cellulitis as well as inflammation of the oviduct and peritonitis.

SHS often implies infections with avian metapneumoviruses. Since infections with avian metapneumoviruses are often complicated by secondary infections with *E. coli*, a sharp distinction might not be possible.

Aetiology

E. coli belongs to the family Enterobacteriaceae; it is a gram-negative, non-spore forming, flagellated, straight rod-shaped bacterium. It measures between 2.0–3.0 × 0.6 µm. Most of the strains are non-haemolytic on blood agar. It is lactose-positive, which sets it apart from other Enterobacteriaceae, and most isolates are motile.

Similar as *Salmonella* spp., it can be serotyped based on its somatic O-antigens, flagellar H-antigens and capsular K-antigens. Of these, the O-antigen is the most important, since the immune response is primarily directed against it. As with *Salmonella*, serogroups are defined based on the O-antigen (Stenutz et al., 2006). It was originally thought that serotypes O1, O2 and O78 were mostly connected with disease; however, many isolates from diseased chickens belong to other serotypes, while not all *E. coli* O1, O2 or O78 are APEC (Blanco et al., 1997).

Identification of APEC is currently based on the detection of a number of virulence genes.

These include genes coding for adhesins responsible for adhesion to the respiratory epithelium, various toxins, protectins that offer protection against the immune system of the host or proteins involved in iron acquisition. None of these genes defines APECs on its own, but usually the genes of several virulence factors cluster together and form pathogenicity islands, which can be considered a defining trait of APECs (Nolan et al., 2013).

Most APECs share virulence with extraintestinal pathogenic *E. coli* (ExPEC), which also include *E. coli* that are pathogenic for humans. This and the possible exchange of virulence genes between APEC and *E. coli* pathogenic for humans has raised concerns that poultry is a reservoir of virulence genes that can make *E. coli* more pathogenic for humans or directly of *E. coli* strains that are pathogenic (Markland et al., 2015).

Pathogenesis and transmission

E. coli is spread vertically as well as horizontally. It is shed in the faeces, which contains about 10^6 colony-forming units (cfu) per gram. The bacteria are spread directly via contaminated faeces, dust, water and on fomites.

Infection takes place orally or by inhalation of dust containing *E. coli*, with the latter being more likely to cause disease. The bacteria multiply in the respiratory tract and can cause inflammation in trachea, lungs or air sacs. There, they enter the blood and spread to other organs, where they also cause inflammations. An alternate route to spread to other organs is within the abdominal air sacs.

E. coli can also be readily isolated from the skin and the feathers. In the skin, *E. coli* can cause cellulitis after penetrating through small injuries like scratches. In 1–day-old chicks, the bacteria can also enter the body through inflamed and insufficiently healed navels (Dho-Moulin and Fairbrother, 1999).

In most disease conditions associated with *E. coli*, it acts as a secondary pathogen. The factors suggested or shown to increase the incidence and severity of *E. coli* infections can be infectious or non-infectious. A comprehensive list is given by Nolan et al. (2013). It comprises more or less all known environmental conditions, management factors and pathogens.

Among the most important non-infectious predisposing factors are high ammonia concentrations in the air that can damage the respiratory epithelium or the skin and thus facilitate the entry of *E. coli*. High ammonia in turn can be related to stocking density, insufficient ventilation, moist litter and the season as well as the presence of further pathogens causing diarrhoea. Furthermore, dusty air is a predisposing factor, since the dust particles serve as vehicles for respiratory *E. coli* infections.

Laying hens kept in alternative systems have more losses due to *E. coli* than layers kept in cages, probably due to increased ammonia concentrations and dust in the air.

The stocking density can also contribute to social stress associated with feather pecking or cannibalism. The stress itself impairs the immune system and thus increases the likelihood of infections with *E. coli*, while cannibalism of the cloacae leads to ascending infections of the reproductive tract.

In addition to these factors, insufficient hygiene, close distances between houses, multiple-age flocks on the farm and short service periods between flocks increase the infection pressure and thus prevalence and severity of *E. coli* infections.

Infections with primary bacterial or viral respiratory pathogens also predispose to more severe infections with *E. coli*, for example by causing damage of the tracheal epithelium, facilitating colonization by *E. coli*. These pathogens include, amongst others, *Ornithobacterium rhinotracheale*, *Mycoplasma gallisepticum*, infectious bronchitis virus (IBV), Newcastle disease virus (NDV) and live vaccines against IBV and NDV. Experimentally, live vaccination with attenuated IBV and NDV can trigger colisepticaemia if birds were *M. gallisepticum* positive (Nakamura et al., 1994). Similarly, infections with enteric parasites like *Ascaridia* spp., coccidia or *Histomonas meleagridis* damage the enteric epithelium and predispose to systemic *E. coli* infection. Infections with immunosuppressive pathogens, especially infectious bursal disease virus (IBDV), can also contribute to a more severe course of *E. coli* infections.

Omphalitis and yolk sac inflammation are also linked to faecal contaminations of the eggshell, delayed egg collection and generally insufficient hygiene of the laying nests, at the hatchery and during transport of eggs and 1–day-old chicks (Dho-Moulin and Fairbrother, 1999).

***E. coli* strains are frequently transmitted vertically from parent flocks to their progeny where they can cause omphalitis and yolk sac inflammation.**

E. coli may spread between the chicks during the hatching and is mostly associated with high mortality rate and inflammation of the yolk sacs. This is mostly due to contamination of the eggshell rather than true vertical transmission inside the egg (Ardrey et al., 1968).

Clinical signs

The various disease conditions caused by *E. coli* can be present in the same flock at the same time and can be caused by identical strains. These conditions are defined by the pathological lesions, but clinical signs also differ between them (Nolan et al., 2013).

Clinical signs of **colisepticaemia** are non-specific and their duration as well as the age of the affected birds can vary. First signs include reduced feed intake and feed conversion. Birds are apathetic and have scrubby feathers. They might retreat from other birds and show laboured breathing without respiratory sounds or coughing. When intervertebral joints are infected, birds show progressive paralysis. Birds can also die peracutely. Morbidity and mortality vary. While morbidity often exceeds 50 %, mortality is usually lower than 5 %.

Symptoms of **coligranulomatosis** are totally non-specific. Birds die, either peracutely or after some time with reduced general condition and weight loss. Mortality may reach 75 %.

Omphalitis and yolk sac inflammation due to *E. coli* are among the most frequent causes of mortality within the first days of life. In acute cases, mortality may reach 10 % within a few days. Chicks and poults can die suddenly without showing clinical signs or show non-specific signs including apathy and decreased intake of feed and water and huddling together under heat sources. They can also show central nervous signs like torticollis, diarrhoea sticking around the cloacae, and laboured breathing. The most specific sign is a reddened and inflamed or blackish and necrotic, swollen navel. Surviving birds will show stunted growth.

As the name suggests, **SHS** is characterised by an oedematous swelling of the skin of the head, especially around the eyes (Fig. 1). Additional signs include conjunctivitis, eye exudate and respiratory sounds. Central nervous signs can be present and some mortality can occur. SHS affects broilers, broiler breeders and layers.

Lesions caused by **coliform cellulitis** are plaques of thickened and hard skin with a dark yellow to brown discolouration and up to several centimetres in diameter. The plaques are mostly located at the lower abdominal region and at the shanks. Affected birds may have a reduced general condition.

Birds suffering an **inflammation of the oviduct** due to *E. coli* infection stop laying eggs and often die.

Post mortem lesions

The most prominent gross lesion of **colisepticaemia** is polyserotitis, especially pericarditis and perihepatitis, characterized by fibrinous material covering the pericardium and the surface of the liver (Fig. 2). Additionally, air sacs are thickened and filled with cheesy exudate (Fig. 3). Spleen,

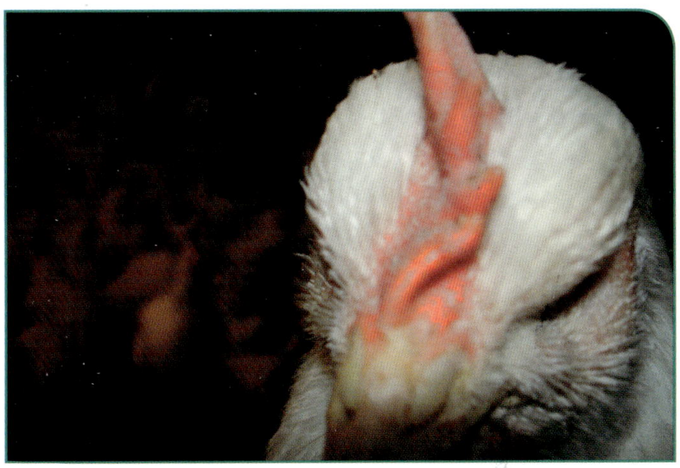

Figure 1. Swollen head.

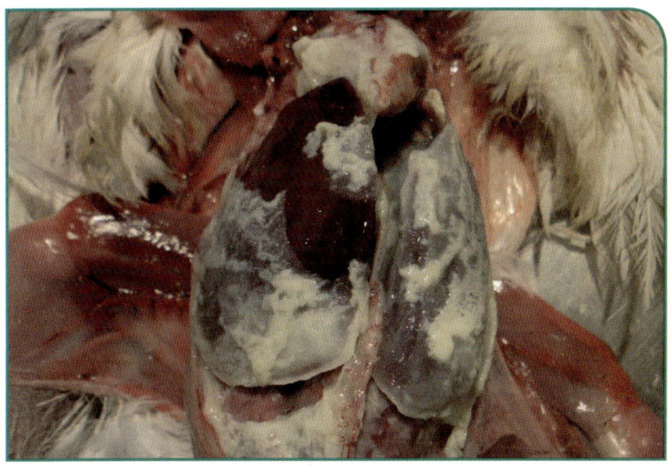

Figure 2. Pericarditis and perihepatitis.

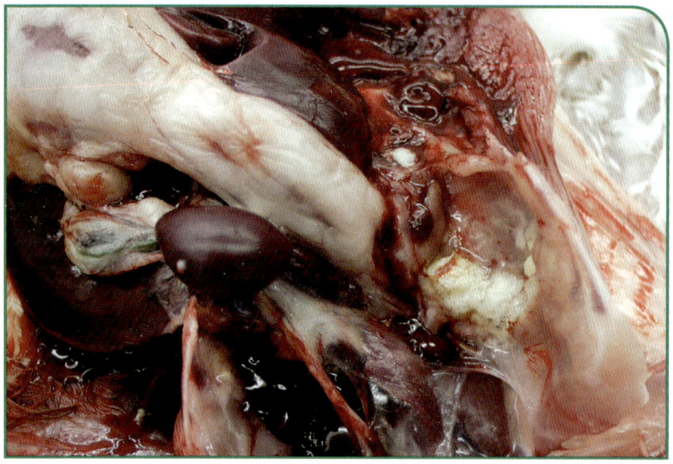

Figure 3. Airsacculitis.

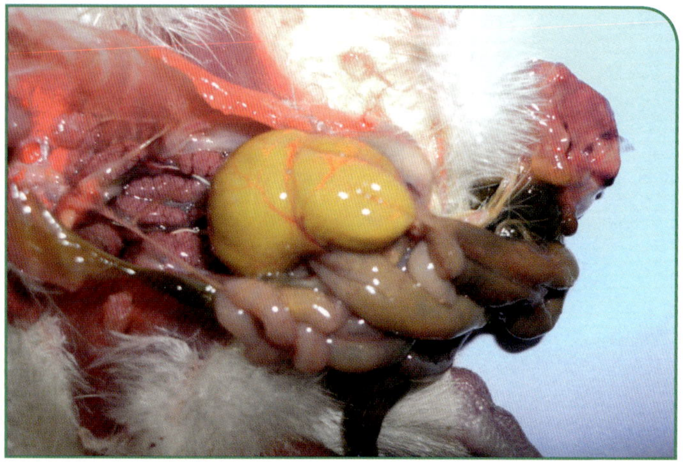

Figure 4. Yolk sac inflammation.

kidneys and liver can also be enlarged. When the infection originated from the respiratory tract, there might be tracheitis and some exudate in the lungs. In cases of chronic respiratory disease (CRD), birds can also show pleuropneumonia. The bacteria can also settle down in the eyes causing panophthalmitis, in the intervertebral joints causing arthritis and in the bones causing osteomyelitis.

Birds with **coligranulomatosis** have typical compact, yellowish granulomas in the mesentery or in the intestinal wall mostly in the caecum. Rarely, there are granulomas in the liver. Microscopically, granulomas consist of a central coagulative necrosis surrounded by few heterophils and giant cells, which develop into typical heterophilic granulomas.

Yolk sac inflammation is characterized by greenish to brownish contents, which are either more fluid than normal or pasty and often has a foul smell (Fig. 4). The blood vessels surrounding the yolk sac, but also in the subcutaneous tissue, are prominently injected. Furthermore, liver, lungs, spleen and kidneys are swollen and dark.

The swelling in **SHS** is caused by accumulation of bloody to fibrinous exudate in the subcutaneous tissue. Additionally, rhinitis and conjunctivitis as well as sinusitis, in some cases, are present. In birds showing central nervous signs, inflammation with fibrinous exudate in the middle ear is present. Histopathologically, there is widespread fibrinoheterophilic inflammation including heterophilic granulomas in the skin and in the cranial bones.

The visible plaques in **coliform cellulitis** cover large areas of serosanguineous or fibrinous exudate in the subcutis mostly close to the cloacae or the thigh (Fig. 5).

Inflamed oviducts are thin-walled, dilated and filled with fibrinous material, which might resemble scrambled eggs. In cases of **peritonitis**, the same material or a milky fluid is present in the body cavity between the internal organs. Usually the ovaries are inflamed as well. The mesenteric vessels are injected.

Diagnostic procedures

Clinical and pathological lesions are non-specific and have to be confirmed by isolation and identification of the bacterium. Generally, isolation of *E. coli* from faeces, organs and swabs does not pose a problem. The bacterium grows on almost all frequently used media, under aerobic as well as under anaerobic conditions at temperatures between 18 °C and 44 °C with an optimum at 37 °C. On blood agar, colonies are round, convex, greyish and smooth. Some *E. coli* strains cause haemolysis. The bacteria stain gram-negative and are straight rods (Fig. 6). The first step in identification can be to check for lactose fermentation on selective media like Endo, Gassner or MacConkey agar. Definite identification requires a full biochemical characterization (Lee and Nolan, 2008).

Isolates can be serotyped for their O-, H- and K-antigens using commercial antisera in the slide agglutination test.

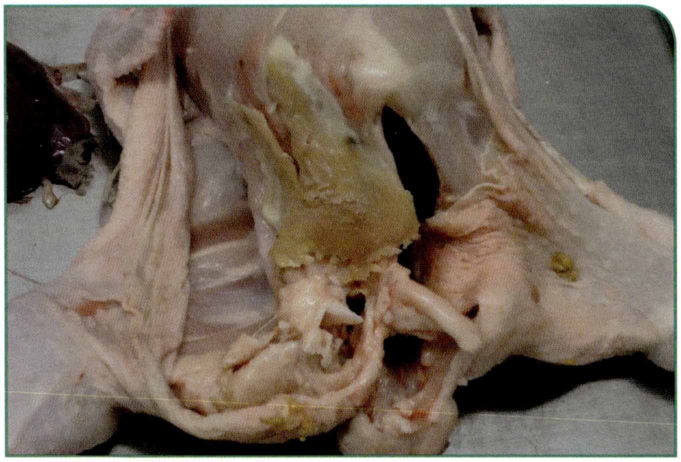

Figure 5. Cellulitis.

PCRs to replace serological determination of the O-antigen have been described (DebRoy et al., 2011). However, the detection of virulence genes, as discussed above, is more relevant than serotyping. For this reason, several multiplex PCR assays have been described and microarray capable to identify a large number of virulence genes on one chip are available (Janßen et al., 2001; Mendonça et al., 2016).

Mixed cultures of different *E. coli* strains are frequent; so, if possible, several colonies should be characterized with the chosen methods. This is especially important if an isolate is used to produce an autogenous vaccine.

Whenever *E. coli* is isolated, it is important to determine if *E. coli* is the primary pathogen or if other bacteria or viruses that are underlying causes of the disease are present.

For this reason and because *E. coli* easily overgrows other bacteria, plates have to be checked so as to not miss those other bacteria. Further measures against *E. coli* overgrowing other bacteria in the case of mixed infections include transporting the samples quickly and cooled and using transport media with a low content of nutrients that support survival but only to a low extent growth of bacteria. Finally, it should be considered that, when the epithelial barrier in the intestinal tract is breaking down at the time of death, *E. coli* can translocate via the bloodstream to other organs. In these cases, isolation of *E. coli* from internal organs would be irrelevant for diagnosis.

The detection of antibodies against *E. coli* using various tests including ELISA is possible; however, due to the ubiquity of the bacterium, results are of limited usefulness.

Treatment

In case of clinical outbreaks, application of antibiotics reducing morbidity and mortality is indicated. Resistances against the most commonly used antibiotics (tetracyclines,

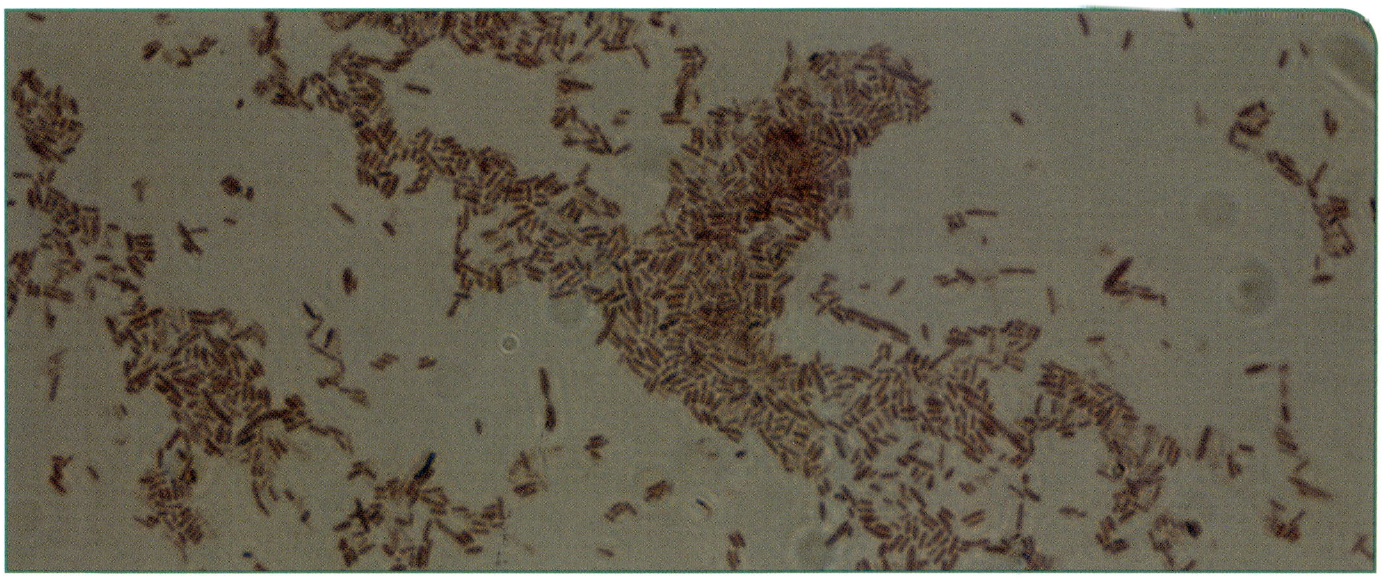

Figure 6. *Escherichia coli* cells. Gram stain.

sulphonamides and aminopenicillins) are frequent, but procedures for antibiotic sensitivity testing are well established and should be done (van den Bogaard et al., 2001; Piccirillo et al., 2014).

Control

Predisposing factors have to be controlled to prevent disease related with *E. coli*. This may include hygienic and management measures to prevent the introduction as well as the spread of infection. Further measures include reducing stress, improving air quality, longer downtimes between flocks combined with thorough cleaning and disinfection.

Since the use of antimicrobials is limited, a vaccine-based approach for the control of avian colibacillosis has obvious benefits (Olsen et al., 2012). Autogenous vaccines against *E. coli* are currently widely used. Inactivated vaccines, sometimes containing more than one *E. coli* serotype, provide protection mostly against challenges with homologous strains. When breeders are vaccinated, their progeny is protected for their first weeks of life.

A subunit vaccine containing fimbrial antigen and flagellar toxin antigen is commercially available in some countries (Gregersen et al., 2010). It protects against most, but not all, *E. coli* strains. Furthermore, a live vaccine for chickens and turkeys, which can be applied by spray or in the drinking water, is on the market. It is a deletion mutant unable to persistently colonize birds or to survive in the environment. The vaccine protected against experimental homologues challenge and has been shown to reduce colibacillosis-like lesions and total mortality and improve other parameters under field conditions (Mombarg et al., 2014).

References

Ardrey WB, Peterson CF and Haggart M. Experimental colibacillosis and the development of carriers in laying hens. *Avian Diseases.* 1968; 12, 505–511.

Blanco JE, Blanco M, Mora A and Blanco J. Production of toxins (enterotoxins, verotoxins, and necrotoxins) and colicins by Escherichia coli strains isolated from septicemic and healthy chickens: relationship with in vivo pathogenicity. *Journal of Clinical Microbiology.* 1997; 35, 2953–2957.

DebRoy C, Roberts E and Fratamico PM. Detection of O antigens in Escherichia coli. *Animal Health Research Reviews.* 2011; 12, 169–185.

Dho-Moulin M and Fairbrother JM. Avian pathogenic Escherichia coli (APEC). *Veterinary Research.* 1999; 30, 299–316.

Gregersen RH, Christensen H, Ewers C and Bisgaard M. Impact of Escherichia coli vaccine on parent stock mortality, first week mortality of broilers and population diversity of E. coli in vaccinated flocks. *Avian Pathology.* 2010; 39, 287–295.

Janßen T, Schwarz C, Preikschat P, Voss M, Philipp H-C and Wieler LH. Virulence-associated genes in avian pathogenic Escherichia coli (APEC) isolated from internal organs of poultry having died from colibacillosis. *International Journal of Medical Microbiology.* 2001; 291, 371–378.

Lee MD and Nolan LK. Colibacillosis. In: A laboratory manual for the isolation, identification and characterization of avian pathogens, L Duforu-Zavala, DE Swayne, JR Glisson, JE Pearson, WM Reed, MW Jackwood, and PR Woolcock, eds. Jacksonville, FA: The American Association of Avian Pathologists. 2008; pp. 10–11.

Markland SM, LeStrange KJ, Sharma M and Kniel KE. Old friends in new places: exploring the role of extraintestinal E. coli in intestinal disease and foodborne illness. *Zoonoses and Public Health.* 2015; 62, 491–496.

Mendonça N, Figueiredo R, Mendes C, Card RM, Anjum MF and da Silva GJ. Microarray evaluation of antimicrobial resistance and virulence of Escherichia coli isolates from Portuguese poultry. 2016; Antibiotics 5.

Mombarg M, Bouzoubaa K, Andrews S, Vanimisetti HB, Rodenberg J and Karaca K. Safety and efficacy of an aroA-deleted live vaccine against avian colibacillosis in a multicentre field trial in broilers in Morocco. *Avian Pathology.* 2014; 43, 276–281.

Nakamura K, Ueda H, Tanimura T and Noguchi K. Effect of mixed live vaccine (Newcastle disease and infectious bronchitis) and Mycoplasma gallisepticum on the chicken respiratory tract and on Escherichia coli infection. *Journal of Comparative Pathology.* 1994; 111, 33–42.

Nolan LK, Barnes HJ, Vaillancourt J-P, Abdul-Aziz TA and Logue CM. Colibacillosis. In: Diseases of Poultry, DE Swayne, JR Glisson, LR McDougald, LK Nolan, DL Suarez, and V Nair, eds. Ames, Iowa: Wiley-Blackwell. 2013; pp. 751–806.

Olsen RH, Christensen H and Bisgaard M. Comparative genomics of multiple plasmids from APEC associated with clonal outbreaks demonstrates major similarities and identifies several potential vaccine-targets. *Veterinary Microbiology.* 2012; 158, 384–393.

Piccirillo A, Giovanardi D, Dotto G, Grilli G, Montesissa C, Boldrin C, Salata C and Giacomelli M. Antimicrobial resistance and class 1 and 2 integrons in Escherichia coli from meat turkeys in Northern Italy. *Avian Pathology.* 2014; 43, 396–405.

Stenutz R, Weintraub A and Widmalm G. The structures of Escherichia coli O-polysaccharide antigens. *FEMS Microbiology Reviews.* 2006; 30, 382–403.

van den Bogaard AE, London N, Driessen C and Stobberingh EE. Antibiotic resistance of faecal Escherichia coli in poultry, poultry farmers and poultry slaughterers. *Journal of Antimicrobial Chemotherapy.* 2001; 47, 763–771.

3 Campylobacteriosis

Infections with thermophilic *Campylobacter* in humans can cause diarrhoea, abdominal pain, vomiting and fever. They further play an indirect role in acute neuromuscular paralysis (Guillain-Barré syndrome). *Campylobacter* spp., especially *C. jejuni*, are the most frequent cause of bacterial gastroenteritis in Europe. In the European Union, the number of diagnosed cases of human campylobacteriosis has exceeded the number of human salmonellosis since at least 2007, and while the case numbers of salmonellosis are decreasing, the yearly numbers of campylobacteriosis tend to increase (EFSA, 2015).

While food derived from other animals, especially cattle, or even vegetables or fruits can be a source of food-borne human campylobacteriosis, contaminated and undercooked poultry and poultry products remain the most important source. The reason is a high prevalence of *Campylobacter* in poultry flocks of up to 100 % depending on climate and management.

In chickens and turkeys, *Campylobacter* spp. are considered part of the normal intestinal flora and *Campylobacter* infections are mostly inapparent.

Aetiology

Campylobacter species belong to the epsilon class of Proteobacteria. The genus *Campylobacter* contains 17 species, four of them have been further divided into eight subspecies (Vandamme and On, 2001). *C. jejuni* and *C. coli* are most frequently encountered in poultry flocks.

***C. jejuni* is responsible for more than 90 % of cases of campylobacteriosis in humans followed by *C. coli*.**

C. lari seems to be more associated with gulls and *C. upsaliensis* with dogs, but both are regarded as primary pathogens in humans. Those four species are often summarily referred to as thermophilic or thermotolerant *Campylobacter*, since their optimal temperature for growth is between 42 °C and 43 °C (Vandamme, 2000).

As their name, which is derived from the Greek word *kampulos* (curved), suggests, *Campylobacter* are comma or corkscrew-shaped bacteria (Vandamme, 2000). They are up to 5 µm long and up to 0.9 µm wide, do not form spores and stain gram-negative (Fig. 1). Their typical rotating movement is due to one or two unipolar or bipolar flagella, which can be up to three times as long as the bacterial cell.

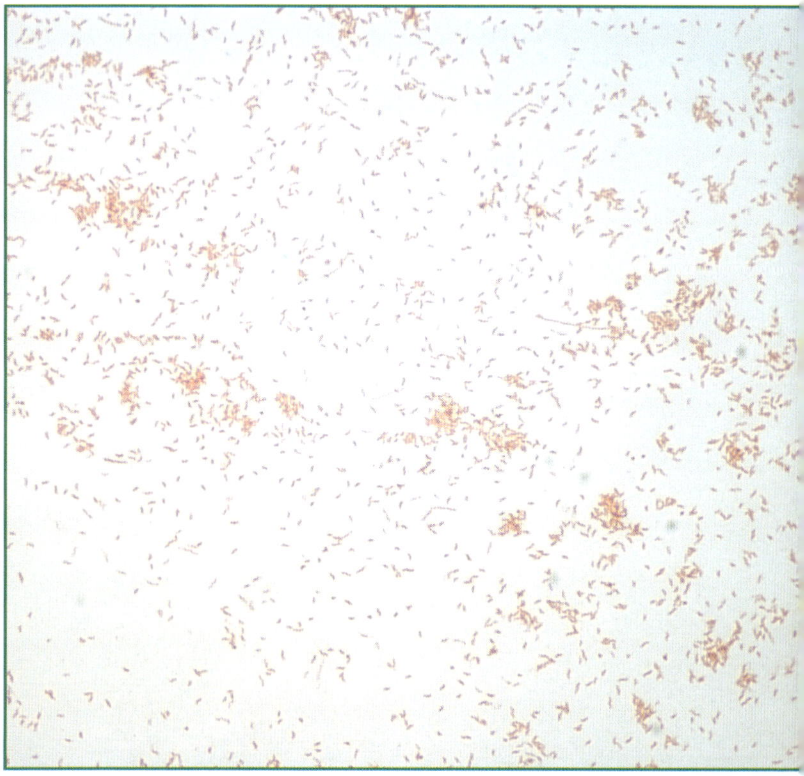

Figure 1. *Campylobacter jejuni* cells. Gram stain. Image courtesy of Dr. Sarah Brüggemann-Schwarze (Institute for Poultry Diseases, Freie Universität Berlin).

Thermophilic *Campylobacter* are fastidious and susceptible to oxidative stress, especially at higher temperatures as well as to low pH. Protected by intestinal content, they can survive outside the host for up to 4 days at 25 °C.

Since they are virtually avirulent for chickens and turkeys, nothing is known about virulence factors for poultry, but a number of putative virulence and toxin genes that may contribute to pathogenicity in human *Campylobacter* infection have been identified (Bolton, 2015).

Pathogenesis and transmission

Horizontal transmission is the most important mode of introduction of *Campylobacter* into poultry flocks. However, the ability of *Campylobacter* to spread is limited by their relatively low tenacity, which can vary between strains. Especially, dry environments kill *Campylobacter* within 1 or 2 hours (Evans and Sayers, 2000).

As with other bacteria, fomites can act as vectors and frequent farm visitors and outside working crews for vaccination or partial depopulation (thinning) are major risk factors.

However, the most important source of introduction of *Campylobacter* is other warm-blooded animals that are infected subclinically and shed the bacteria in their faeces.

Most notably, these include, but are not limited to, other feed producing livestock like cattle and swine, pets like dogs and cats, pests like rats and mice as well as wild birds. Insects, especially darkling beetles and flies, can be mechanical vectors (Hald et al., 2008; Sommer et al., 2013).

Furthermore, drinking water plays a central role in the spread of the bacteria within an infected flock, persistence on the farm and to a lesser extent introduction of *Campylobacter*. Protected by biofilms in water pipes and even unprotected in cool water, *Campylobacter* can survive for several weeks, and dirty bell drinkers or cups under nipple drinkers also serve as a reservoir that readily infects drinking birds. *Campylobacter* are also associated with protozoa in the drinking water, which also confers protection (Sahin et al., 2002).

Vertical transmission of *Campylobacter* spp. seems possible, since *Campylobacter* are capable to penetrate the eggshell and have been isolated from the inside and outside of eggs, and their DNA has been detected by PCR in newly hatched chickens (Newell and Fearnley, 2003). On the other hand, the bacteria usually survive only for a limited time in embryonated eggs and cause high embryo mortality. Thus, vertical transmission does not play a major role in the spread of *Campylobacter*. This is also demonstrated by the fact that only very rarely *Campylobacter* are isolated from flocks younger than 2 weeks of age, even though this is also explained by the protection offered by maternal antibodies (Hafez et al., 2001; Newell and Fearnley, 2003).

It is not uncommon to detect several *Campylobacter* genotypes in the same flock, at the same time or at different ages. Besides, the same strains are often encountered in several houses on the farm or in consecutive flocks. Both facts indicate the relative ease of horizontal introduction of *Campylobacter* into flocks as well as the existence of reservoirs on the farm or nearby (Sahin et al., 2015).

After oral infection, *Campylobacter* colonize the intestines, most importantly caeca and colon. Shedding in faeces, where their concentration can reach up to 10^9 cfu/g, is usually limited in time, but just as whole flocks the individual bird can quickly become infected with another genotype. In tendency, younger birds are more often infected with *C. jejuni*, which has the ability to spread more quickly within a flock, while older birds are more often infected with *C. coli*, which colonizes birds for a longer time (El-Adawy et al., 2012).

Campylobacter cells remain in the mucus layer of the intestinal crypts and usually do not adhere to host cells or invade them, even though they have been isolated from spleen and liver. The host mounts an effective immune response and may even clear infection if given enough time.

While circulating antibodies are probably not protective, maternal antibodies, which are transferred from the yolk sac to the intestines, protect chickens during the first 2 to 3 weeks of their live (Sahin et al., 2015).

Clinical signs and post mortem lesions

In rare cases, if young birds that are not protected by maternal antibodies are infected with *Campylobacter*, they can develop diarrhoea, show slower growth and even increased mortality. Gross lesions are mild and may include watery intestinal contents or hyperaemia of the caecal wall. Histologically, diffuse lymphoplasmacellular mucosal infiltration of the mucosa with inflammatory cells as well as thickening, shortening, and fusion of villi in the ileum have been observed. Not all *Campylobacter* strains seem to be capable to induce disease, even in susceptible birds (Van Deun et al., 2008).

Avian vibrionic hepatitis is, as the name suggests, a liver disease caused by vibrionic bacteria, i.e. bacteria morphologically similar to *Campylobacter*. The disease caused necrosis and inflammation in the liver and was prevalent in layer flocks in the 1960s. Since then, for unknown reasons the disease has been observed very rarely and a characterization of the isolated gram-negative, curved, rod-shaped bacteria is lacking (Jennings et al., 2011).

Diagnostic procedures

The best sample for isolation of *Campylobacter* is caecal content, although faeces can also be suitable. Due to the low tenacity of *Campylobacter*, samples should be transported as quickly as possible and cooled to the laboratory. Brucella broth, Cary-Blair medium and Stuart medium, each with various modifications, have been shown to be suitable transport media (Bai et al., 2014).

Procedure for the isolation of thermophilic *Campylobacter* is described in detail in ISO 10272. Similar to the isolation of *Salmonella* spp., the isolation of *Campylobacter* is done in several steps. Since *Campylobacter* are fastidious and require rich media, selectivity of liquid and solid media is achieved by adding various antibiotics like polymixin B, rifampicin, trimethoprim and/or cycloheximid.

Campylobacter in samples can be enriched in liquid media like Preston broth or Bolton broth. Preston broth might be superior to Bolton broth but can also favour the growth of *C. coli* over *C. jejuni*. Both media contain lysed blood; the use of horse blood will give better results compared to sheep blood. Cultures in Bolton broth are incubated for 2–4 hours at 37 °C first followed by 24–48 hours incubation at 42 °C; cultures in Preston broth are incubated for 24–48 hours at 42 °C from the beginning. If sealed tubes are used, there is no need for a microaerophilic atmosphere.

From the liquid medium, the organisms are transferred onto selective bacterial plates, usually containing blood and activated charcoal-like Karmali agar or modified charcoal with cefoperazone deoxycholate agar (mCCDA). The plates are incubated for 24–48 hours at 42 °C under microaerophilic conditions. Differences between the various media seem to be minor. Colonies are smooth, colourless or transparent or light cream and convex or flat. Their size can vary between pin-point to several millimetres in diameter, but are usually 1–2 mm (Fig. 2). *Campylobacter* are oxidase positive.

For biochemical identification, suspect colonies need to be subcultured on blood agar. Reactions that vary between species and have been used for species identification include catalase reaction, hippurate hydrolysis and indoxyl acetate test (Table 1). Since resistance of *C. coli* and *C. jejuni* against fluoroquinolones is increasing, resistance against nalidixic acid should not be relied on any more to differentiate these two species from *C. lari* and *C. upsaliensis*.

Because the biochemical tests are unreliable and take some time, a large number of multiplex PCR assays have been developed and validated to identify *Campylobacter* spp.

Depending on their sensitivity, they can also be applied for direct detection of pathogens from samples or from the enrichment broth (Wang et al., 2002; Josefsen et al., 2004; He et al., 2010).

For epidemiological investigations, isolates can be typed. Serotyping by haemagglutination has been described, but the method is labour-intensive and requires a large number of antisera. Furthermore, cross-reactions are common. Current methods routinely used are typing by

Table 1. Differentiation characters of thermophilic *Campylobacter* spp. (modified from Kaplan and Weissfeld, 1994).

CRITERIA	*C. JEJUNI*	*C. COLI*	*C. LARI*	*C. UPSALIENSIS*
Catalase test	+	+	+	-
Nalidixic acid	Sensitive	Sensitive	Resistant/Sensitive	Sensitive
Cefalotin	Resistant	Resistant	Resistant	Sensitive
Metronidazole	M	+	+	M
Hippurate hydrolysis	+	-	-	-
Indoxyl acetate hydrolysis	+	+	-	+
H_2S/TSI	-	F	-	-
2.0 % NaCl	-	-	M	-
Growth on minimal medium	-	+	-	-
Sodium fluoride	+	+	+	-
$KMnO_4$	+	+	F	F
0.02 % safranin	+	+	+	F

F: 14–50 % strains positive; M: 60–93 % strains positive; TSI: triple sugar iron.

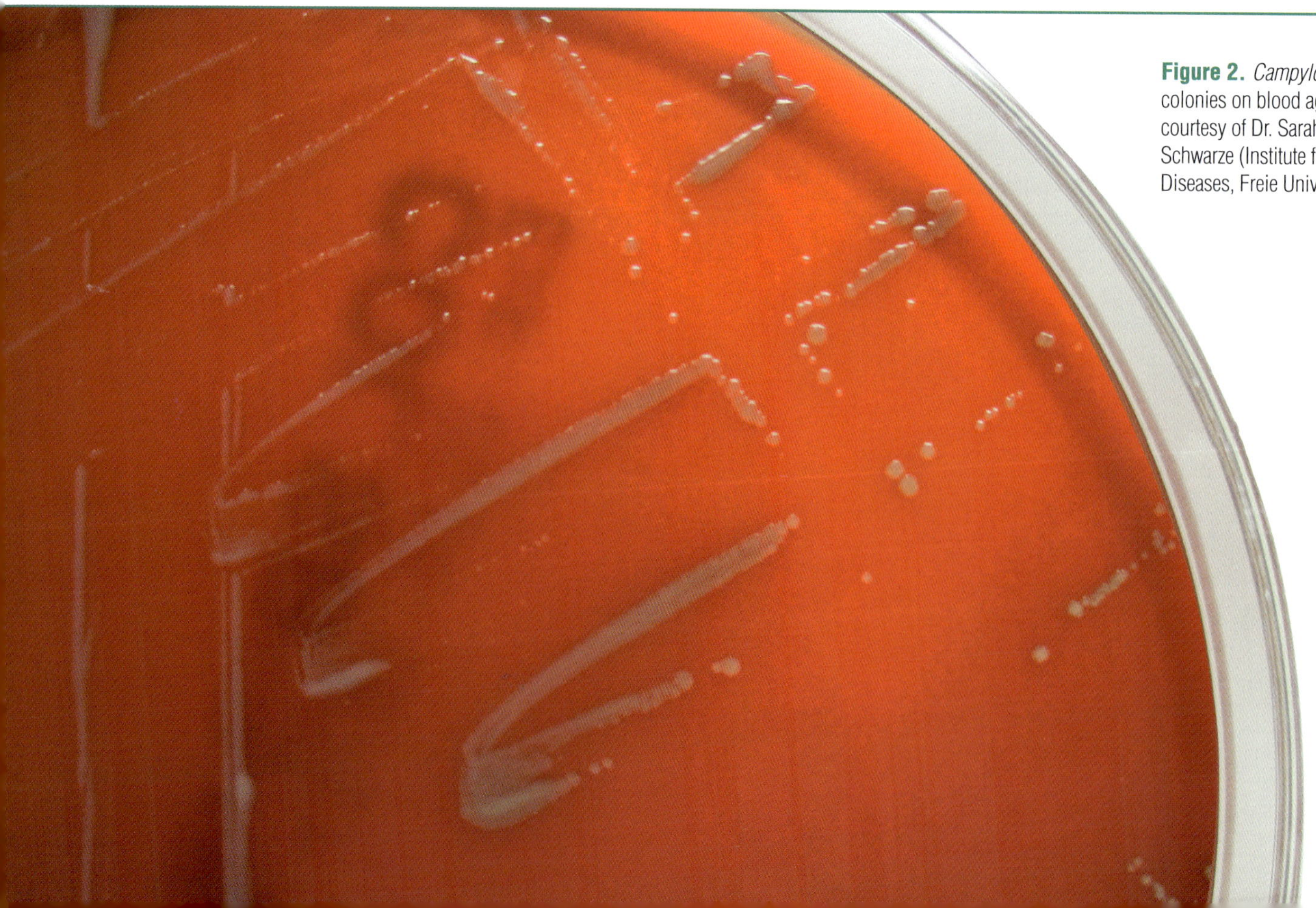

Figure 2. *Campylobacter jejuni* colonies on blood agar. Image courtesy of Dr. Sarah Brüggemann-Schwarze (Institute for Poultry Diseases, Freie Universität Berlin).

macrorestriction followed by pulsed-field gel electrophoresis (PFGE), sequencing the short variable region of the flaA gene as well as multilocus sequence typing (MLST). For *C. jejuni*, a microarray assay for characterization is commercially available (Lévesque et al., 2008; El-Adawy et al., 2013).

Under hostile environmental conditions like a lack of nutrients, extreme pH or temperature or drying, thermophilic *Campylobacter* become viable but non-culturable (VNC). Although VNC stage *Campylobacter* cannot be cultivated using bacteriological methods, they still can infect humans and animals. Isolation in embryonated chicken eggs is also possible (Oliver, 2005; Klančnik et al., 2009).

Treatment

Treatment of thermophilic *Campylobacter* infections in poultry is not indicated due to their lack of virulence for chickens and turkeys.

Control

Since farm visitors and the presence of other animals on the farm are the major risk factors for introduction of *Campylobacter* into a farm, prevention by improving biosecurity should put an emphasis on these aspects. Fly screens were also highly efficient to decrease the prevalence of *Campylobacter*-positive flocks. Water pipes and drinkers need to be kept clean. Chlorinating the drinking water or the addition of organic acids as well as organic acids in the feed can reduce colonization of birds by *Campylobacter* (Chaveerach et al., 2004; Heres et al., 2004). The use of competitive exclusion or probiotics has yielded inconsistent results (Sahin et al., 2015).

Dry bedding in poultry houses will help to limit the spread of the bacteria within a flock. Feed, good gut health, litter material, as well as heating and ventilation in turn are factors to keep litter drier. Additionally, under experimental conditions, acidifying the litter with aluminum sulfate or sodium bisulfate reduced *Campylobacter* colonization frequency and populations in the ceaca, but the effect wears off as the pH in the litter increases again (Line, 2002; Line and Bailey, 2006).

There are no commercial vaccines available. Experimentally, attenuated *C. jejuni* strains used as vaccine did not colonize the birds long enough to induce protection. On the other hand, vaccination with recombinant *Salmonella* expressing *Campylobacter* antigen can reduce colonization (Sahin et al., 2015).

Finally, treatment of birds with bacteriophages against *Campylobacter* can reduce *Campylobacter* counts in the intestines. However, even if mixtures containing several phages are used, resistance rates of bacteria are high and resistances quickly develop (Fischer et al., 2013).

References

Bai Y, Cui SH, Xu X and Li FQ. Modification and evaluation of Brucella broth based *Campylobacter jejuni* transport medium. *Biomedical and Environmental Sciences* (BES). 2014; 27, 466–470.

Bolton DJ. Campylobacter virulence and survival factors. *Food Microbiology*. 2015; 48, 99–108.

Chaveerach P, Keuzenkamp DA, Lipman LJA and Knapen FV. Effect of organic acids in drinking water for young broilers on Campylobacter infection, volatile fatty acid production, gut microflora and histological cell changes. *Poultry Science*. 2004; 83, 330–334.

EFSA. The European Union summary report on trends and sources of zoonoses, zoonotic agents and food-borne outbreaks in 2013. *EFSA Journal*. 2015; 13, 3991.

El-Adawy H, Hotzel H, Tomaso H, Neubauer H and Hafez HM. Elucidation of colonization time and prevalence of thermophilic Campylobacter species during turkey rearing using multiplex polymerase chain reaction. *Poultry Science*. 2012; 91, 454–459.

El-Adawy H, Hotzel H, Tomaso H, Neubauer H, Taboada EN, Ehricht R and Hafez HM. Detection of genetic diversity in *Campylobacter jejuni* isolated from a commercial turkey flock using flaA typing, MLST analysis and microarray Assay. *PLOS ONE*. 2013; 8, e51582.

Evans SJ and Sayers AR. A longitudinal study of campylobacter infection of broiler flocks in Great Britain. *Preventive Veterinary Medicine*. 2000; 46, 209–223.

Fischer S, Kittler S, Klein G and Glünder G. Impact of a single phage and a phage cocktail application in broilers on reduction of *Campylobacter jejuni* and development of resistance. *PLOS ONE*. 2013; 8, e78543.

Hafez HM, Schroth S, Stadler A and Schulze D. Detection of Salmonella, Campylobacter and verotoxin producing *E. coli* in turkey flocks during rearing and processing. *Archive Für Geflügelkunde*. 2001; 65, 130–135.

Hald B, Skovgård H, Pedersen K and Bunkenborg H. Influxed insects as vectors for *Campylobacter jejuni* and *Campylobacter coli* in Danish broiler houses. *Poultry Science*. 2008; 87, 1428–1434.

He Y, Yao X, Gunther NW, Xie Y, Tu S-I and Shi X. Simultaneous detection and differentiation of *Campylobacter jejuni*, *C. coli*, and *C. lari* in chickens using a multiplex real-time PCR assay. *Food Analytical Methods*. 2010; 3, 321–329.

Heres L, Engel B, Urlings HAP, Wagenaar JA and van Knapen F. Effect of acidified feed on susceptibility of broiler chickens to intestinal infection by Campylobacter and Salmonella. *Veterinary Microbiology*. 2004; 99, 259–267.

Jennings JL, Sait LC, Perrett CA, Foster C, Williams LK, Humphrey TJ and Cogan TA. Campylobacter jejuni is associated with, but not sufficient to cause vibrionic hepatitis in chickens. *Veterinary Microbiology*. 2011; 149, 193–199.

Josefsen MH, Jacobsen NR and Hoorfar J. Enrichment followed by quantitative PCR both for rapid detection and as a tool for quantitative risk assessment of food-borne thermotolerant campylobacters. *Applied and Environmental Microbiology*. 2004; 70, 3588–3592.

Kaplan R and Weissfeld AS. Campylobacter, Helicobacter, and related organisms. In: Clinical and Pathogenic Microbiology, BJ Howard, J Keiser, T Smith, AS Weissfeld and RC Tilton, eds. St. Louis: Mosby. 1994; pp. 453–460.

Klančnik A, Guzej B, Jamnik P, Vučković D, Abram M and Možina SS. Stress response and pathogenic potential of *Campylobacter jejuni* cells exposed to starvation. *Research in Microbiology*. 2009; 160, 345–352.

Lévesque S, Frost E, Arbeit RD and Michaud S. Multilocus sequence typing of *Campylobacter jejuni* isolates from humans, chickens, raw milk, and environmental water in Quebec, Canada. *Journal of Clinical Microbiology*. 2008; 46, 3404–3411.

Line JE. Campylobacter and Salmonella populations associated with chickens raised on acidified litter. *Poultry Science*. 2002; 81, 1473–1477.

Line JE and Bailey JS. Effect of on-farm litter acidification treatments on Campylobacter and Salmonella populations in commercial broiler houses in northeast Georgia. *Poultry Science*. 2006; 85, 1529–1534.

Newell DG and Fearnley C. Sources of Campylobacter colonization in broiler chickens. *Applied and Environmental Microbiology*. 2003; 69, 4343–4351.

Oliver JD. The viable but nonculturable state in bacteria. *Journal of Microbiology*. 2005; 43, 93–100.

Sahin O, Morishita TY and Zhang Q. Campylobacter colonization in poultry: sources of infection and modes of transmission. *Anim. Health Res. Rev. Conf. Res. Work. Anim. Dis.* 2002; 3, 95–105.

Sahin O, Kassem II, Shen Z, Lin J, Rajashekara G and Zhang Q. Campylobacter in poultry: ecology and potential interventions. *Avian Diseases*. 2015; 59, 185–200.

Sommer HM, Heuer OE, Sørensen AIV and Madsen M. Analysis of factors important for the occurrence of Campylobacter in Danish broiler flocks. *Preventive Veterinary Medicine*. 2013; 111, 100–111.

Van Deun K, Pasmans F, Ducatelle R, Flahou B, Vissenberg K, Martel A, Van den Broeck W, Van Immerseel F and Haesebrouck F. Colonization strategy of *Campylobacter jejuni* results in persistent infection of the chicken gut. *Veterinary Microbiology*. 2008; 130, 285–297.

Vandamme P. Taxonomy of the family Campylobacteraceae. In: CAMPYLOBACTER, I Nachamkin and MJ Blaser, eds. Washington, DC: American Society Microbiolgy. 2000; pp. 3–26.

Vandamme P and On SL. Recommendations of the subcommittee on the taxonomy of Campylobacter and related bacteria. *International Journal of Systematic and Evolutionary Microbiology*. 2001; 51, 719–721.

Wang G, Clark CG, Taylor TM, Pucknell C, Barton C, Price L, Woodward DL and Rodgers FG. Colony multiplex PCR assay for identification and differentiation of *Campylobacter jejuni*, *C. coli*, *C. lari*, *C. upsaliensis*, and *C. fetus* subsp. fetus. *Journal of Clinical Microbiology*. 2002; 40, 4744–4747.

4 Fowl cholera

Fowl cholera is a highly contagious disease caused by infection with *Pasteurella multocida*. The disease can take two different courses: (a) peracute/acute septicaemia characterized by high morbidity or (b) chronic infection characterized by localized abscesses or pneumonia. Fowl cholera occurs sporadically and has a worldwide distribution. *P. multocida* can infect a very wide range of birds and mammals and fowl cholera has been described in a large variety of birds.

The disease has a long history, having been described first in the late 18th century. The bacterium was isolated 100 years later by its name patron Louis Pasteur (Fig. 1), and it was with this bacterium in chickens that he discovered the concept of the attenuation of pathogens by passage *in vitro*.

Aetiology

P. multocida is a gram-negative staining, rod-shaped bacterium, about 0.2–0.4 by 0.6–2.5 μm in size (Fig. 2). It is cytochrom c oxidase positive, non-motile and does not form spores. Presence or absence of a capsule has consequences for virulence and colony morphology as discussed in connection with pathogenesis and diagnosis.

The species *P. multocida* can be divided into three subspecies: *P. multocida* ssp. *multocida*, *P. multocida* ssp. *septica* and *P. multocida* ssp. *gallicida*. These subspecies have been defined based on DNA homology, but also differ in their ability to use various sugars (Mutters et al., 1985). All these subspecies can cause fowl cholera, but *P. multocida* ssp. *multocida* is most frequently encountered in chickens

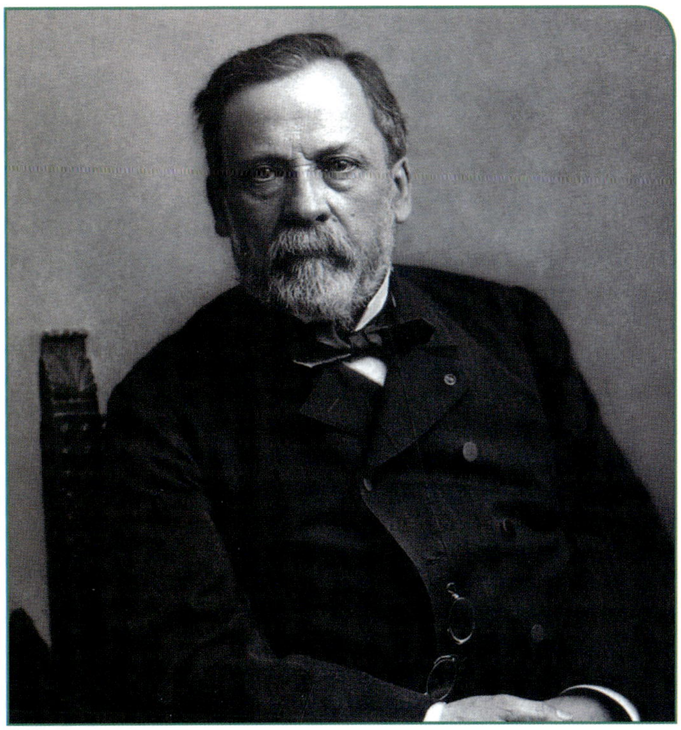

Figure 1. Louis Pasteur (1822–1895). Image extracted from Wikimedia Commons.

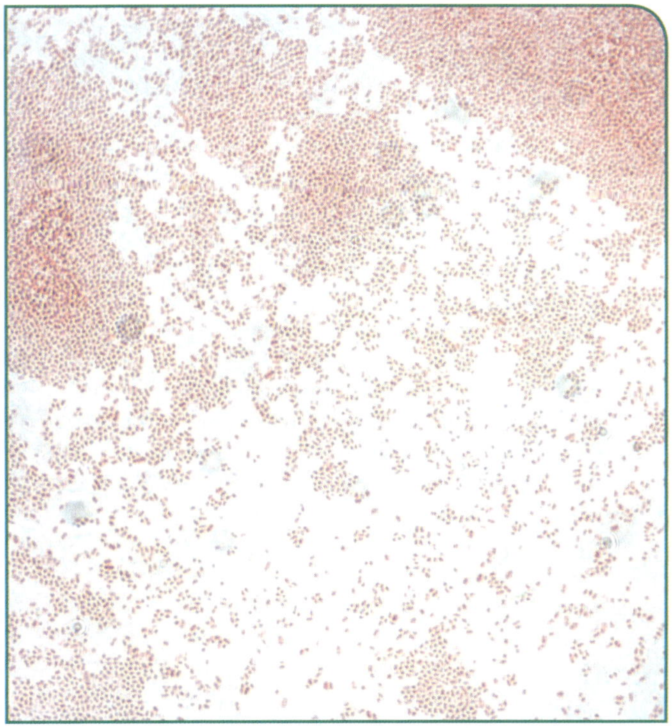

Figure 2. *Pasteurella multocida* cells. Gram stain. Image courtesy of Dr. Sarah Brüggemann-Schwarze (Institute for Poultry Diseases, Freie Universität Berlin).

and turkeys, while *P. multocida* ssp. *gallicida* is mostly associated with waterfowl (Christensen et al., 2014).

The antigenic formula of an isolate is given as capsular and somatic antigen. Five different capsular types designated by letters A, B, D, E and F and 16 somatic antigens designated by numbers 1–16 are known. Traditionally, capsular types A and F have been associated with poultry, but in recent years types B and D have also been isolated from birds. The most frequently isolated serovar from fowl cholera outbreaks in birds is serovar A. Most somatic serotypes were isolated from birds except serotypes 8 and 13 (Christensen et al., 2009). The prevalence of a certain serotype seems more correlated to the geographical region than to the host. Serotypes do not correlate with the subspecies or phenotype.

In the environment, *P. multocida* is susceptible to acidity, dryness and warmer temperatures. Depending on these factors, it can survive in soil between less than 1 week and up to 4 months. After outbreaks, the environment does not seem to harbour infective bacteria for more than 2 weeks. *P. multocida* is easily destroyed by ordinary disinfectants, sunlight, drying, or heat.

Pathogenesis and transmission

While all kinds of fomites might be the source of introduction of *P. multocida* into poultry flocks, other animals infected with the bacterium are more significant. Especially wild birds are regarded as the most important vectors.

P. multocida can also infect many different mammals and causes important diseases in cattle, sheep and pigs like haemorrhagic septicaemia, bronchopneumonia or atrophic rhinitis. However, high virulent strains for cattle and sheep are apathogenic for poultry. It can also infect these species commensally and is considered part of the normal bacterial flora in the oral cavity of cats and dogs.

On the other hand, strains isolated from pigs, cats, mice and sparrows have been shown to be highly pathogenic for poultry and they must be considered as a potential source of infection in poultry flocks.

While isolates of *P. multocida* may be capable to infect more than one host species, virulence for one species is not linked with virulence for another, even though some virulence genes are not host specific (Furian et al., 2016). Thus, mammals, including humans, can harbour isolates of *P. multocida* that are capable to cause fowl cholera.

The role of insects in the spread of *P. multocida* seems to be minor. Under experimental conditions, flies, in contrast to the red fowl mite, transmitted the disease, but in practice separation of groups by poultry netting was able to stop the spread of the disease in the presence of a large number of flies (Glisson et al., 2013). In addition, *P. multocida* survives long enough to be spread by contaminated crates, feed bags, shoes, and other equipment. There is no indication of vertical transmission of *P. multocida*. Under field conditions, it has been almost impossible to ascertain the mode of introduction of the infection into a flock.

The mucous membranes of the upper respiratory tract, including the conjunctivae, are the most important route of infection. From there, the infection can spread along the respiratory system to lungs and air sacs or to the air spaces of the cranial bone, the middle ear and the brain.

On the other hand, isolation of *P. multocida* from peritoneum and oviduct as well as cloacae indicates that other mucosal membranes may serve as ports of entry (Christensen et al., 2009).

Virulent strains can enter the blood, probably facilitated by mucosal macrophages (Matsumoto et al., 1991). Virulence is enhanced by the production of a capsule, which can contain components that help invasion, but not all isolates with a capsule are virulent. While endotoxins and protein toxins can contribute to virulence and various virulence genes have been described, granulocytes battling the infection might cause much of the damage in fowl cholera (Wilkie et al., 2012).

Infected birds shed *P. multocida* from the beak, nose and conjunctiva, but very rarely in the faeces (cloacal carriers). If birds survive an infection, they can stay chronically infected, especially in the choanae and the nasal cavity.

These birds continue shedding the bacterium for an indefinite amount of time.

Another route of infection is through skin injuries. This is especially relevant after bites by carnivores like dogs, cats or racoons. Non-specific wound infections due to *P. multocida* are also caused by isolates that do not cause fowl cholera (Derieux, 1978).

Clinical signs

Besides the widely varying virulence of the infecting strain, the severity of disease after infection with *P. multocida* depends on species and age of the host.

Generally, turkeys, ducks and geese are more susceptible than chickens, and older birds are more susceptible than younger ones.

Mortality in turkey flocks is often higher than 50 %, while losses in chickens do not usually exceed 20 %. On the other hand, an impressive field outbreak of fowl cholera involving a contaminated vaccine caused mortality between 30 % and 90 % in laying hens older than 16 weeks compared to no mortality in pullets (Hungerford, 1968).

In the case of peracute or acute fowl cholera, beside sudden deaths, infected birds can show largely non-specific signs like depression, ruffled feathers, fast breathing, coughing, sneezing as well as nasal, ocular and oral mucous discharge, but also watery and whitish and later greenish diarrhoea. They usually die a few hours after the onset of these signs, but can still recover.

If the disease turns chronic or is caused by *P. multocida* with lower virulence, signs are, in addition to the above mentioned non-specific signs, consequences of localized inflammations. They include dyspnoea and/or respiratory sounds, if the respiratory tract is infected, conjunctivitis, as well as swollen wattles, combs or snouts, sinuses or joints of the legs or wings. Infections of the middle ear or meninges lead to torticollis (Fig. 3).

Post mortem lesions

As the clinical signs, pathological lesions vary between the acute and chronic course of the disease. In some cases, an intermediate form with acute and chronic lesions can be observed. In acute cases, post mortem lesions are characterized by hyperaemia and include congested vessels and haemorrhages in and on a variety of organs like pericardium or abdominal fat. In some cases, additionally the liver is swollen with visible necrotic foci. The crop and intestines may be filled with mucus. In active laying hens, the ovary is inflamed, hyperaemic and with flaccid or ruptured follicles. Microscopic lesions are disseminated intravascular coagulation (DIC) and bacteria in the blood vessels and heterophilic infiltrations in liver, lungs and other parenchymatous organs.

Chronic cases are characterized by fibrinous inflammation easily recognizable by the firm, caseous exudate. Since most infections happen via the respiratory tract, consequently affected organs include trachea, air sacs and lungs (Figs. 4 and 5), sinuses and pneumatic bones as well as the cranial bones, meninges and the middle ear.

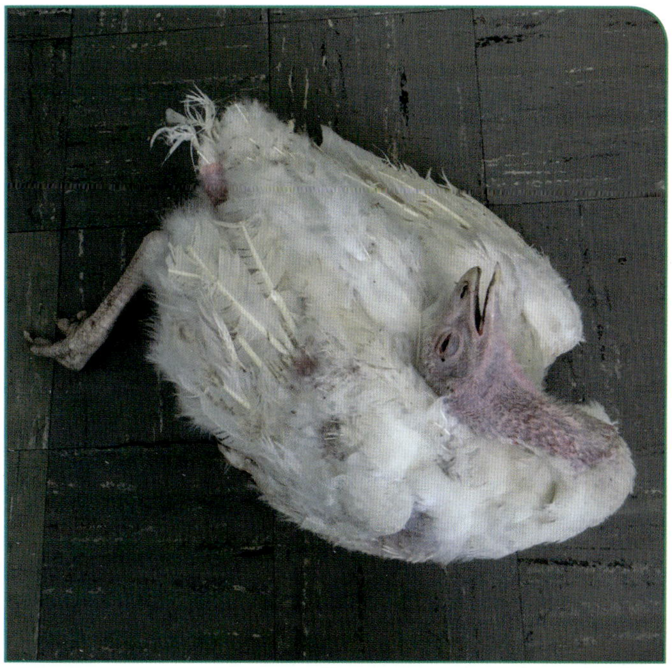

Figure 3. Turkey hen with torticollis due to otitis media in a case of fowl cholera. Image courtesy of Dr. Manuela Crispo (California Animal Health and Food Safety Laboratory System, Turlock branch).

In turkeys, lesions are generally localized in the lungs and include oedema and uni- or bilateral consolidation of the lungs with fibropurulent exudate.

Other affected organs may include joints (Fig. 6), liver, oviduct and body cavity, especially in the case of egg peritonitis after the rupture of follicles. Microscopically, the lesions consist of necrosis, accumulation of fibrin and heterophilic infiltrations. Multinuclear giant cells can also be present.

Diagnostic procedures

A presumptive diagnosis based on clinical signs and post mortem lesions can be quickly hardened by preparing blood smears or imprints of inflamed lungs and staining them with methylene blue, which is also a component of Wright's stain. *P. multocida* will stain characteristically bipolar (Fig. 7).

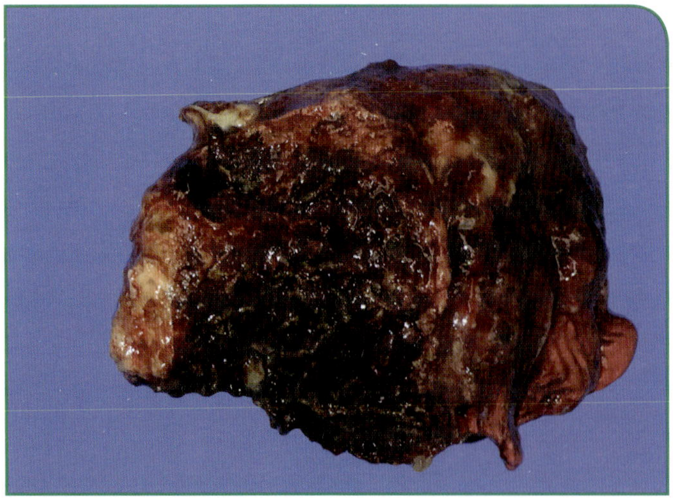

Figure 4. Subacute pneumonia in a case of fowl cholera in turkeys. Note dark red colour indicating hyperaemia. Image courtesy of Dr. Manuela Crispo (California Animal Health and Food Safety Laboratory System, Turlock branch).

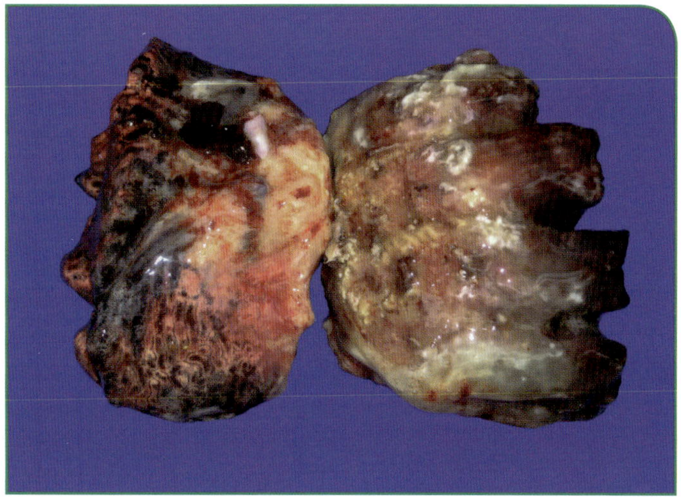

Figure 5. Chronic fibrinous pneumonia in a case of fowl cholera in turkeys. Image courtesy of Dr. Manuela Crispo (California Animal Health and Food Safety Laboratory System, Turlock branch).

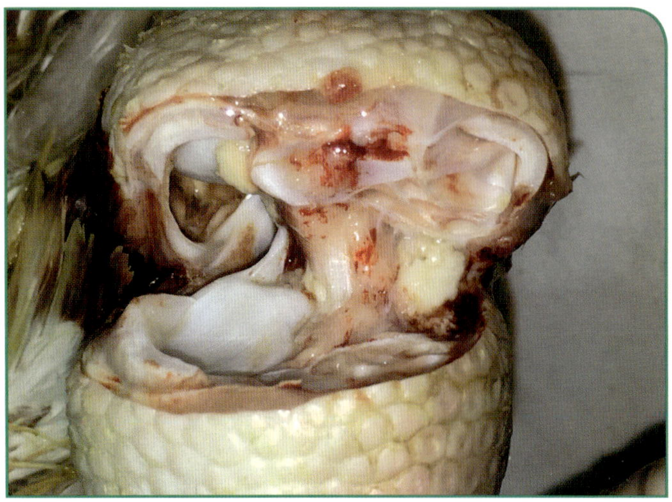

Figure 6. Tenosynovitis in a case of fowl cholera in turkeys. Image courtesy of Dr. Manuela Crispo (California Animal Health and Food Safety Laboratory System, Turlock branch).

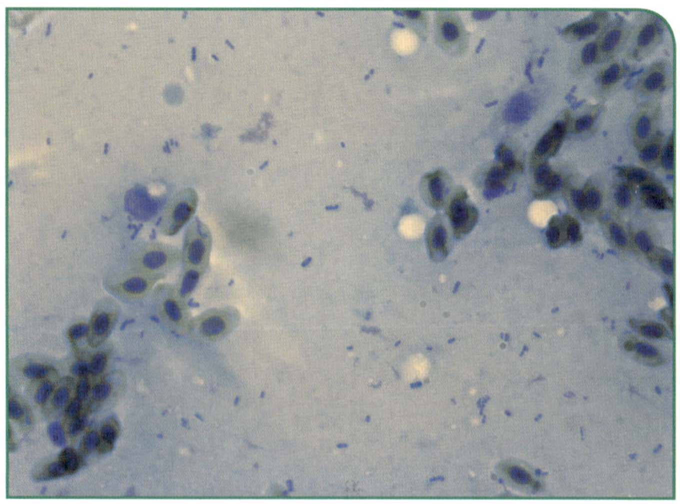

Figure 7. *Pasteurella multocida* cells in blood smear with methylene blue stain. Note bipolar appearance.

For confirmation of the diagnosis, the bacterium can be easily isolated from all infected organs including heart blood and bone marrow in acute cases.

Species identification as *P. multocida* can be done by routine biochemical characterization.

Choanal swabs are the preferred sample for isolation from living birds, for example to identify chronically infected but healthy carriers.

Dextrose starch agar containing 5 % chicken serum or blood agar are the preferred media. While serum from some animals, most notably horses and sheep, can inhibit growth of *P. multocida* on dextrose starch agar, *P. multocida* will also grow on sheep blood agar. It will not grow on MacConkey agar. Growth should be visible after incubation at 37 °C for 18–24 hours under aerobic or anaerobic conditions (Glisson et al., 2013). Colony morphology of *P. multocida* is variable and to some extent dependent on the host. Colonies of chicken isolates are circular with a diameter of up to 3 mm, smooth, convex and without haemolysis (Fig. 8). Colonies are iridescent and sectored when viewed with oblique illumination or, more rarely, blue with or without some degree of iridescence. Iridescence is only shown by isolates with capsules. If an isolate with iridescent colonies is passaged repeatedly and loses its capsule, colonies of later passages will look blue. Since there is some correlation between the presence of a capsule and virulence, this property of *P. multocida* colonies also allows some conclusions about the virulence of the isolate (Hughes, 1930).

As the bacteria in organs smears, cells from fresh isolates will stain bipolar, while cells from isolates that have been passaged multiple times will not.

Several PCR assays for identifying isolated *P. multocida* or detecting *P. multocida* directly in clinical samples have been described, e.g. by Corney et al. (2007).

Traditionally, serotyping was done by passive haemagglutination assay for the capsular antigen and by tube agglutination test or agar gel diffusion test for the somatic antigen (Heddleston et al., 1972). Today, PCR assays that are specific of a certain capsular type are more common. Besides the lack of need for specific antisera, a major advantage is that these PCRs can also type isolates that have lost their capsule during passaging. PCRs for somatic typing have also been described (Townsend et al., 2001; Harper et al., 2015).

For epidemiological purposes, a variety of methods have been adapted to *P. multocida*. These include electrophoretic separation of outer membrane proteins, restriction enzyme analysis in combination with pulsed-field gel electrophoresis (PFGE), random amplification of polymorphic DNA, multilocus sequence typing (MLST) and others. These and further methods have been reviewed by Dziva et al. (2008).

For detection of antibodies against *P. multocida*, an ELISA is commercially available. It is of little value in diagnosing on-going outbreaks, but is useful for surveillance.

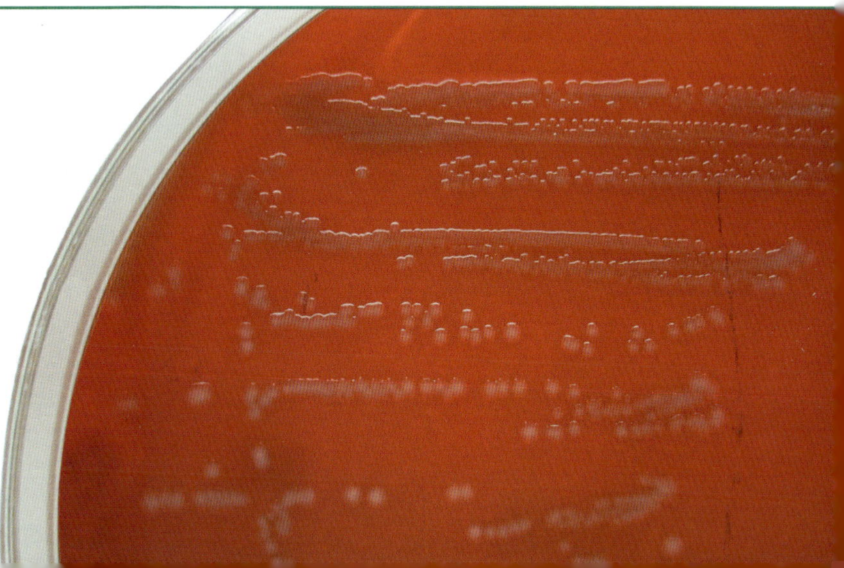

Figure 8. *Pasteurella multocida* colonies on blood agar. Image courtesy of Dr. Sarah Brüggemann-Schwarze (Institute for Poultry Diseases, Freie Universität Berlin).

Treatment

The treatment of *P. multocida* infections is very difficult because different strains have variable susceptibilities to antibiotics. The sensitivity pattern depends on the source of the strain and the routinely used drugs in an area. Thus, an investigation of the sensitivity pattern of the isolated strain is necessary for successful treatment. Another problem related to fowl cholera treatment is the route of medication application; if the flocks are recumbent and not able to drink the medicated water, a single bird injection with antibiotics should be used (Hafez et al., 1992).

Reduction of mortality and morbidity has been achieved by treatment with sulphonamides, tetracyclines, erythromycin, fluoroquinolones and streptomycin. Even though *P. multocida* is a gram-negative bacterium, treatment with penicillin is also effective. *P. multocida* has lower resistance rates than related bacteria, but antimicrobial resistance testing is still advisable (Jones et al., 2013).

The success of treatment with antibiotics depends on an early diagnosis and start of treatment. If treatment begins too late or if the antibiotic is given at subtherapeutic doses, acute outbreaks will turn chronic.

Treatment should continue as long as the withdrawal time allows, since mortality is likely to return after the end of medication. Treatment of chronic cases is usually not satisfactory, probably because the antibiotics do not reach the bacteria in the abscesses.

Control

For preventing introduction of *P. multocida* into poultry flocks, flocks should be strictly separated from other farm animals and protected from wild birds and rodents. Multiple-age farms are at increased risk, since older birds are likely to be subclinically infected carriers and can infect younger flocks.

If fowl cholera is endemic, vaccination can be tried. Live attenuated as well as inactivated vaccines against *P. multocida* are licensed in some countries.

Live vaccines have the advantage that they induce protection against heterologous serotypes, partly because *P. multocida* seems to produce more immunogenic proteins *in vivo* than *in vitro*. For best protection, chickens should be vaccinated by wing-web or subcutaneously, while turkeys can be vaccinated orally. On the downside, even though the vaccine strains are attenuated, they have retained a relatively high virulence and can cause chronic fowl cholera and significant mortality, which sometimes needs to be treated with antibiotics. If possible, treatment with antibiotics should be avoided until at least 4 days post-vaccination when the vaccine has induced at least a partial immunity (Olson and Schlink, 1986).

Inactivated vaccines contain isolates of several somatic serotypes and will only protect against homologous challenges. Bacterins usually contain whole cells of serotypes 1, 3, and 4 emulsified in an oil adjuvant. In case of problems with isolates of other serotypes, autogenous vaccines can be used. Specific vaccination programmes have been discussed by Glisson et al. (2013).

References

CHRISTENSEN H, KUHNERT P, NØRSKOV-LAURITSEN N, PLANET PJ AND BISGAARD M. Family Pasteurellaceae. In: The Prokaryotes: Gammaproteobacteria, Stackebrandt E, Rosenberg E, Delong E, Steven L and Thompson F, eds. New York: Springer. 2014; pp. 535–564.

CHRISTENSEN JP, BOJESEN AM AND BISGAARD M. Fowl Cholera. In: Poultry Diseases, Pattison M, McMullin PF, Bradbury JM and Alexander DJ, eds. Noida: Elsevier. 2009; pp. 149–154.

CORNEY BG, DIALLO IS, WRIGHT LL, HEWITSON GR, JONG AJD, BURRELL PC, DUFFY PF, STEPHENS CP, RODWELL BJ, BOYLE DB AND BLACKALL PJ. *Pasteurella multocida* detection by 5' Taq nuclease assay: A new tool for use in diagnosing fowl cholera. *Journal of Microbiological Methods*. 2007; 69, 376–380.

DERIEUX WT. Response of young chickens and turkeys to virulent and avirulent *Pasteurella multocida* administered by various routes. *Avian Diseases*. 1978; 22, 131–139.

DZIVA F, MUHAIRWA AP, BISGAARD M AND CHRISTENSEN H. Diagnostic and typing options for investigating diseases associated with *Pasteurella multocida*. *Veterinary Microbiology*. 2008; 128, 1–22.

FURIAN TQ, BORGES KA, LAVINIKI V, DA SILVEIRA ROCHA SL, DE ALMEIDA CN, DO NASCIMENTO VP, SALLE CTP AND DE SOUZA MORAES HL. Virulence genes and antimicrobial resistance of *Pasteurella multocida* isolated from poultry and swine. *Brazilian Journal of Microbiology*. 2016; 47, 210–216.

GLISSON JR, HOFACRE C AND CHRISTENSEN JP. Fowl Cholera. In: Diseases of Poultry, DE Swayne, JR Glisson, LR McDougald, LK Nolan, DL Suarez and V Nair, eds. Ames, Iowa: Wiley-Blackwell. 2013; pp. 807–823.

HAFEZ H, EMELE J AND KRUSE W. *Pasteurella-multocida* infection in turkey - review and experience in turkey farms. *Archiv für Geflügelkunde*. 1992; 56, 45–52.

HARPER M, JOHN M, TURNI C, EDMUNDS M, ST. MICHAEL F, ADLER B, BLACKALL PJ, COX AD AND BOYCE JD. Development of a rapid multiplex PCR assay to genotype *Pasteurella multocida* strains by use of the lipopolysaccharide outer core biosynthesis locus. *Journal of Clinical Microbiology*. 2015; 53, 477–485.

HEDDLESTON KL, GALLAGHER JE AND REBERS PA. Fowl cholera: gel diffusion precipitin test for serotyping *Pasteurella multocida* from avian species. *Avian Diseases*. 1972; 16, 925–936.

HUGHES TP. The epidemiology of fowl cholera II. Biological properties of *P. avicida*. *Journal of Experimental Medicine*. 1930; 51, 225–238.

HUNGERFORD TG. A Clinical Rate on Avian Cholera; The Effect of Age on the Susceptibility of Fowls. *Australian Veterinary Journal*. 1968; 44, 31–32.

JONES KH, THORNTON JK, ZHANG Y AND MAUEL MJ. A 5-year retrospective report of *Gallibacterium anatis* and *Pasteurella multocida* isolates from chickens in Mississippi. *Poultry Science*. 2013; 92, 3166–3171.

MATSUMOTO M, STRAIN JG AND ENGEL HN. The fate of *Pasteurella multocida* after intratracheal inoculation into turkeys. *Poultry Science*. 1991; 70, 2259–2266.

MUTTERS R, IHM P, POHL S, FREDERIKSEN W AND MANNHEIM W. Reclassification of the genus *Pasteurella* Trevisan 1887 on the basis of deoxyribonucleic acid homology, with proposals for the new species *Pasteurella dagmatis*, *Pasteurella canis*, *Pasteurella stomatis*, *Pasteurella anatis*, and *Pasteurella langaa*. *International Journal of Systematic and Evolutionary Microbiology*. 1985; 35, 309–322.

OLSON LD AND SCHLINK GT. Onset and duration of immunity and minimum dosage with CU cholera vaccine in turkeys via drinking water. *Avian Diseases*. 1986; 30, 87–92.

TOWNSEND KM, BOYCE JD, CHUNG JY, FROST AJ AND ADLER B. Genetic organization of *Pasteurella multocida* cap Loci and development of a multiplex capsular PCR typing system. *Journal of Clinical Microbiology*. 2001; 39, 924–929.

WILKIE IW, HARPER M, BOYCE JD AND ADLER B. *Pasteurella multocida*: Diseases and Pathogenesis. In: *Pasteurella multocida*, Aktories K, Orth JHC and Adler B, eds. Springer Berlin Heidelberg. 2012; pp. 1–22.

5 *Ornithobacterium rhinotracheale* infection

Ornithobacterium rhinotracheale (ORT) is incriminated as causative agent in the respiratory disease complex. Infections with ORT alone or in combination with other pathogens cause an acute and highly contagious disease of chickens and turkeys. The disease is accompanied by heavy economic losses, by increased mortality rates, increased medication costs, increased condemnation rates due to aerosacculitis and drops in egg production. The infection has been recognized in many countries worldwide.

Aetiology

ORT is a gram-negative, rod-shaped to pleomorphic, fastidious and slow-growing, non-motile, non-sporulating bacterium (Fig. 1). The genus *Ornithobacterium* is a member of the Flavobacteriaceae within the Cytophaga-Flavobacterium-Bacteroides phylum and represents a rather distinct line of descent within this family.

ORT lacks pili, fimbriae and plasmids. Most strains (90–95 %) of ORT are resistant to gentamicin and polymyxin. All isolates produce oxidase; however, some isolates are cytochrome oxidase negative. In addition, all isolates are β-galactosidase (ONPG) positive as well as indole and catalase negative. Tests with variable results include urease and gelatinase reaction as well as the p-nitrophenyl-beta-D-glucoside (PNPG) test (Hafez and Vandamme, 2011).

ORT has been isolated from many different gallinaceous bird species like chicken, turkey, guinea fowl, pheasant, partridge, quail and chukar as well as from duck, goose, pigeon, gull, ostrich, rook and birds of prey.

Currently, 18 serotypes designated A to R are known. However, there is no indication of any host specificity of the serotypes. The prevalence of the serotypes is dependent on the host and the geographic region and may change over time. Currently, most of the chicken isolates belong to the serotype A, while the turkey isolates are more heterogeneous and belong to serotypes A, B, C, D and E. Within this bacterial species, isolates with different virulence seem to exist. Neither the origin nor the serotype of the ORT strains does have an effect on the pathogenicity (Chin et al., 2013).

Pathogenesis and transmission

The disease is spread horizontally by direct and indirect contact through aerosols or drinking water. Infection takes place by the respiratory route and the bacterium is shed in respiratory secretions. It is possible that wild birds play a role in the dissemination of the bacterium.

Vertical transmission is suspected, since some research has isolated ORT at very low incidence from reproductive organs and hatching eggs, infertile eggs and dead embryos. However, it is not yet known if this vertical transmission is caused by ovarian or cloacal contamination (Gornatti Churria et al., 2012).

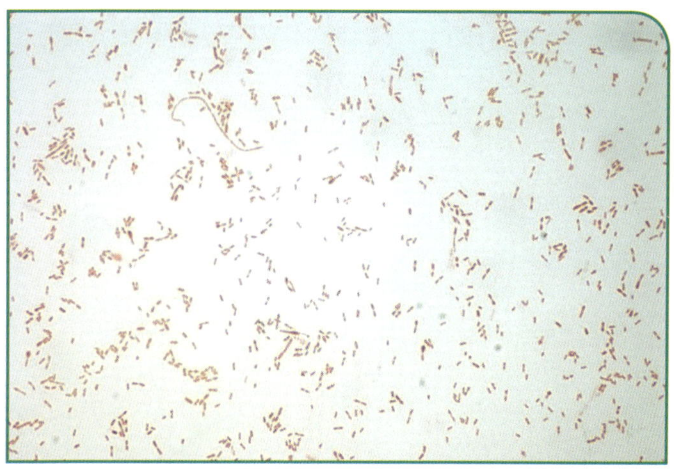

Figure 1. ORT is a gram-negative, rod-shaped to pleomorphic and non-sporulating bacterium (Gram stain).

There is very little information about pathogenesis. The bacterium has been detected in various organs, but infection is mostly restricted to the upper and lower respiratory tract. No virulence factors are known.

Clinical signs

The severity of clinical signs, duration of the disease and mortality are extremely variable and are influenced by many environmental factors such as poor management, inadequate ventilation, high stocking density, poor litter conditions, poor hygiene, high ammonia level, concurrent diseases and the type of secondary infection. In most field cases, especially in chickens, in which ORT is detected, other respiratory pathogens like Newcastle disease virus (NDV), infectious bronchitis virus (IBV), turkey rhinotracheitis (TRT), *Bordetella* spp., *Escherichia coli* (*E. coli*) as well as *Chlamydophila psittaci* (*C. psittaci*) are present. There are many reports showing synergism between ORT and those pathogens under experimental conditions (Marien et al., 2005, 2007; Chin et al., 2013).

Turkeys outbreaks have been mostly observed in male birds over 14 weeks of age. However, in many cases young poults between the 2nd and 8th week of age could also be found to be affected. The mortality ranges between 1–15 % during the acute phase, approximately 8 days. Initial symptoms are coughing, sneezing and nasal discharge, followed in some cases by severe respiratory distress, dyspnoea, prostration, sinusitis (Fig. 2) and arthritis. The symptoms are accompanied with a reduction in feed consumption and water intake. In turkey breeder flocks, clinical signs are mostly accompanied with drops in egg production of 2–5 % and increases in the number of unsettable hatching eggs (van Empel and Hafez, 1999).

Clinical signs in broilers generally appear between the 3rd and 4th week of age with a mortality rate of 2–10 % (Hauck et al., 2015).

The clinical signs are depression, decrease in food intake, reduced weight gains, transit nasal discharge, sneezing, followed by facial oedema. In **broiler breeders and layers** the disease primarily affects the birds at the peak of production, mostly between 24th and 52nd week of age. The first signs are mild respiratory symptoms. The mortality is variable and relatively low in uncomplicated cases. The symptoms are generally accompanied with a drop in egg production, decrease in egg size and poor eggshell quality. Fertility and hatchability are unaffected in many cases (van Empel and Hafez, 1999).

Post mortem lesions

Pathological lesions are more severe when other respiratory pathogens are present and more common in turkeys than in chickens.

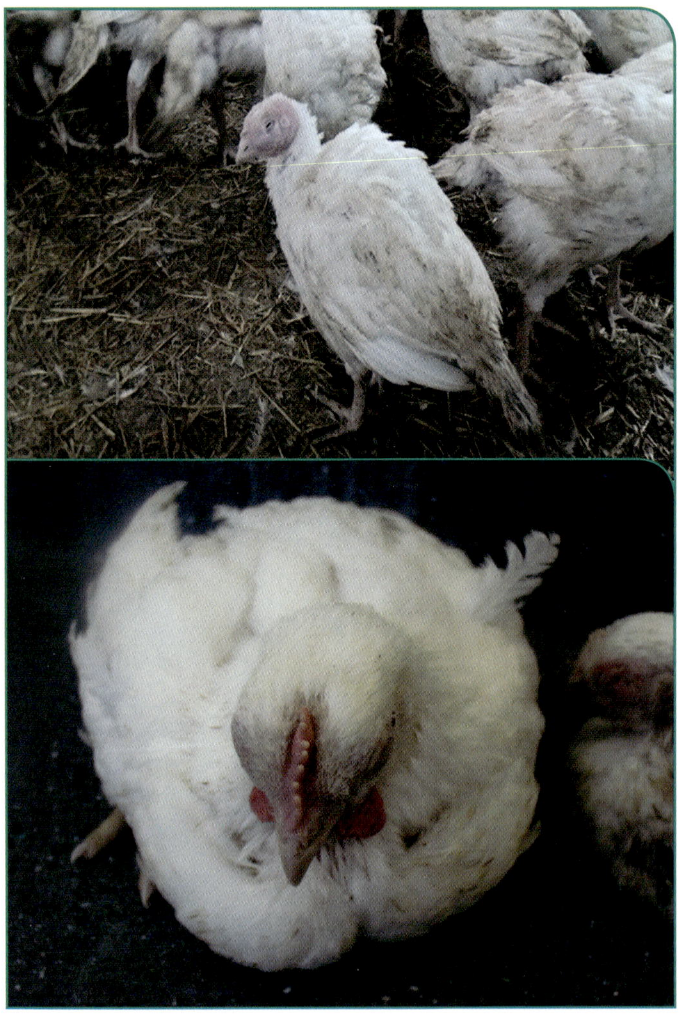

Figure 2. Sinusitis.

The lesions in broilers include pneumonic lungs, pleuritis and airsacculitis.

In the air sac, accumulation of creamy, "yoghurt-like" exudate can mostly be detected. In turkeys, lesions are generally localized in the lungs, and include oedema and uni- or bilateral consolidation of the lungs with fibrinopurulent exudate (Fig. 3) as well as caseous or fibrinous exudate in the air sacs (Fig. 4), airsacculitis, peritonitis and enteritis could be detected. In some cases, conjunctivitis, arthritis (Fig. 5), meningitis and inflammation of the cranial bones associated with ORT have been described.

The most common histopathological lesions in the infraorbital sinus and trachea are heterophilic or mononuclear inflammatory cell infiltration. In the lungs and air sacs, inflammation was characterized by heterophilic infiltration and/or fibrin accumulation (Hauck et al., 2015).

Diagnostic procedures

Clinical signs and lesions are of little value in diagnosis, since many other conditions produce similar clinical signs and post mortem lesions. Accurate diagnosis must be substantiated by direct detection or isolation of the causative bacteria and/or indirectly through detection of antibodies using serological examination (Fig. 6).

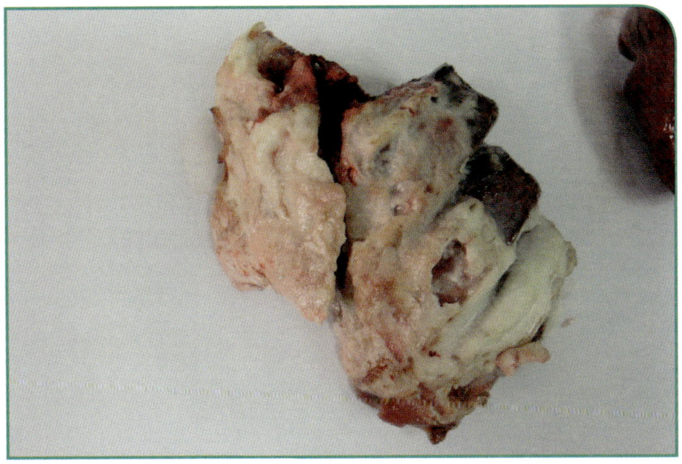

Figure 3. Lungs with fibrinopurulent exudate.

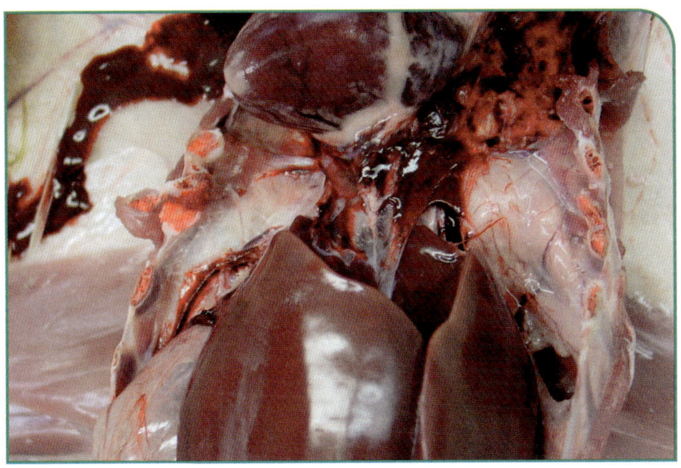

Figure 4. Fibrinous exudate in the air sacs.

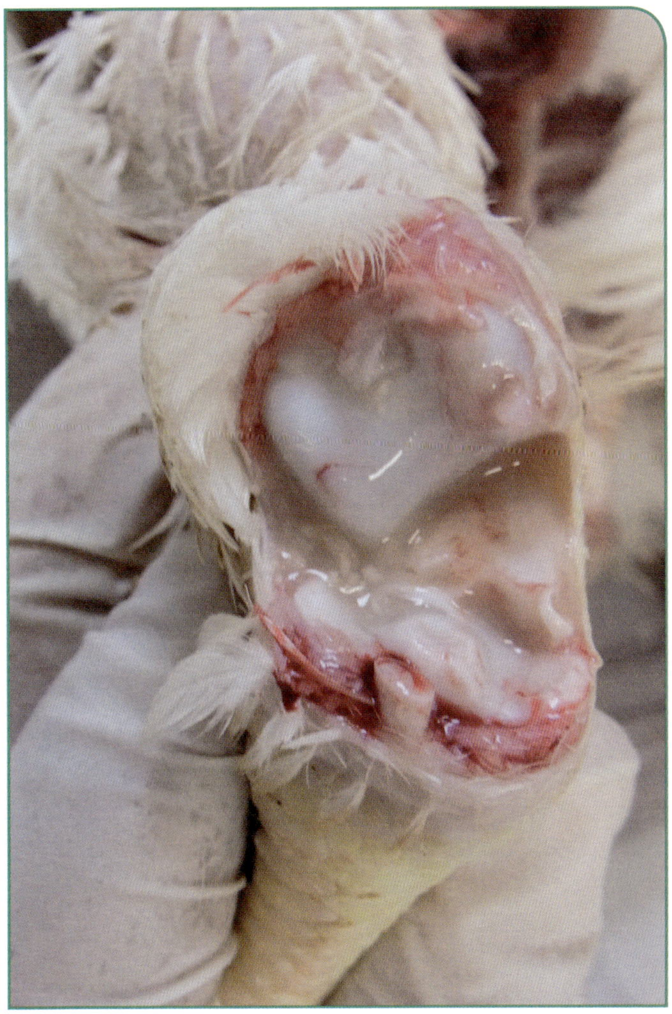

Figure 5. Arthritis.

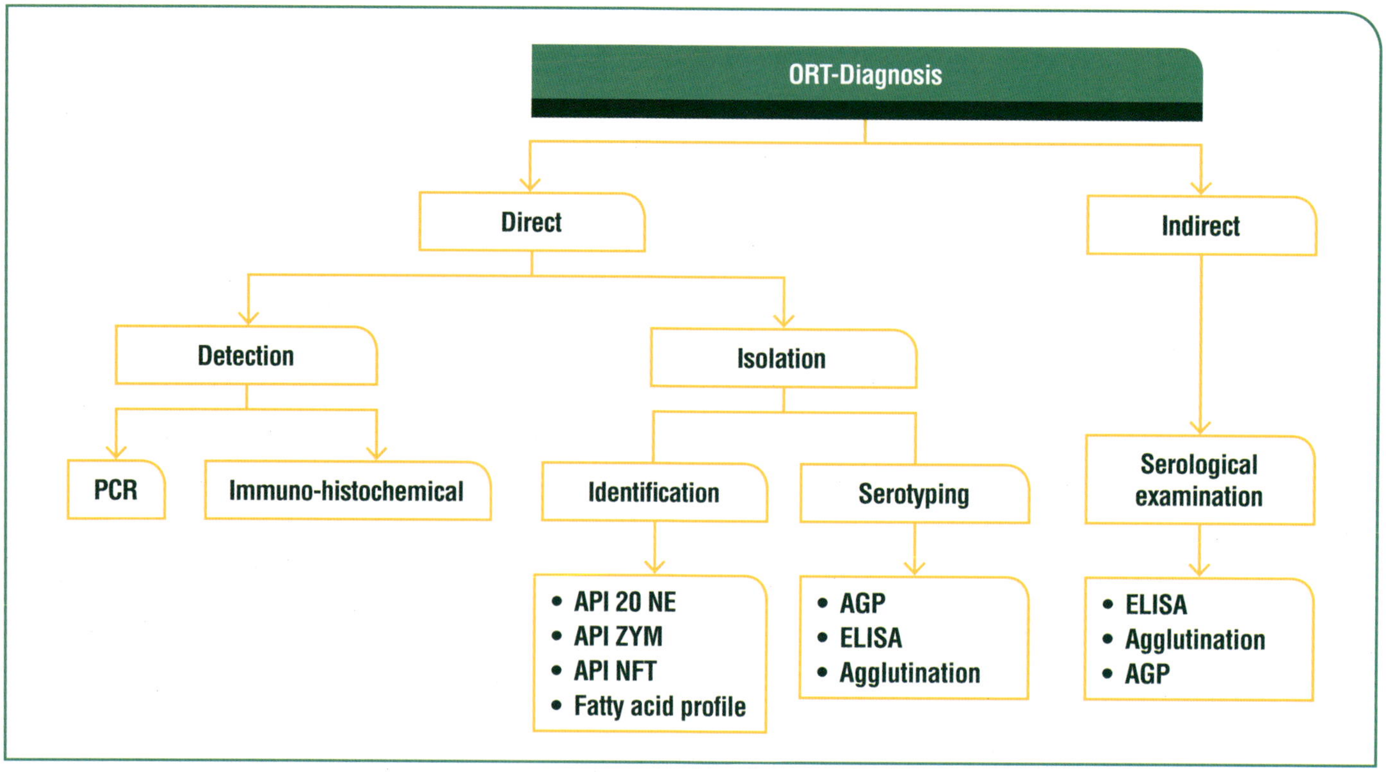

Figure 6. Scheme for diagnosis of infections with ORT.

For detection of the bacteria a sensitive immuno-histochemical staining or a specific polymerase chain reaction (PCR) can be performed (Hafez, 1998).

Samples for bacterial isolation should be collected at an early stage of the disease. ORT can usually be isolated from trachea, lungs, air sacs and sinus. Swabs should be shipped cooled and in transport medium. Differences between various transport media like Amies gel medium and Stuart gel medium in keeping ORT alive are minor (Numee et al., 2012). Blood agar with 5–10 % sheep blood is commonly used for primary isolation, but ORT can also grow on tryptone soy agar and chocolate agar. No growth on MacConkey agar, Endo agar, Gassner agar, Drigalski litmus lactose agar, and Simmons citrate media. More often than not, ORT occurs in mixed culture with other bacteria, especially *E. coli.* A good selective medium for culturing ORT is not yet available. The addition of 0.5 µm/ml gentamicin and 0.5 µm/ml polymyxin to the sheep blood media may suppress contaminating bacteria, but also the growth of some ORT strains. The incubation of the plates at 37 °C for 48 hours under anaerobic or microaerobic conditions is recommended, but ORT may grow under aerobic conditions. Colonies are very small, grey to grey-white and non-haemolytic (Fig. 7) (van Empel and Hafez, 1999; Chin et al., 2013).

Serotyping is done using heat extracted antigen and reference hyperimmune sera by agar gel precipitation test (AGP) or enzyme-linked immunosorbent assay (ELISA). However, AGP is the method of choice for serotyping. Indirect diagnosis for detection of antibodies can be carried out using serological examination as slide agglutination test using antigen prepared from different serotypes or ELISA. The method of choice for detection of antibodies against ORT is the ELISA. The serotype specificity of the ELISA depends on the method of antigen extraction used for coating the ELISA plates. Commercially available ELISA kits are able to detect antibodies against all tested ORT serotypes (Hafez and Sting, 1999).

Treatment

The treatment of infections with antibiotics is very difficult because of the inconstant and regional sensitivity of ORT strains to antibiotics. For example, most of turkey isolates from Germany and the Netherlands are resistant to enrofloxacin, while isolates from other countries are sensitive against enrofloxacin. It is advisable to test the sensitivity of every isolate. However, currently there is no standard method, and accurate breakpoints to classify isolates as susceptible or resistant are missing.

Under field conditions, water medication, using amoxicillin at a dose level of 250 ppm for 3–7 days, has given satisfactory results. Application of chlortetracycline at a dose level of 500 ppm in drinking water for 4–5 days also appeared to be very effective (Marien et al., 2007).

Control

ORT infections appear to have become endemic and can affect every newly restocked flock even in previously cleaned and disinfected houses. This is especially true in areas with intensive poultry production as well as in multiple-age farms. There also seems to be a high prevalence in backyard flocks. Failure to clean and disinfect properly after an infected flock has left can cause infection of neighbouring flocks, and the causative agent can cycle continuously from house to house.

Proper cleaning and disinfection of the houses between flocks is important to minimize the infection pressure.

Figure 7. Typical morphology of ORT colonies on blood agar.

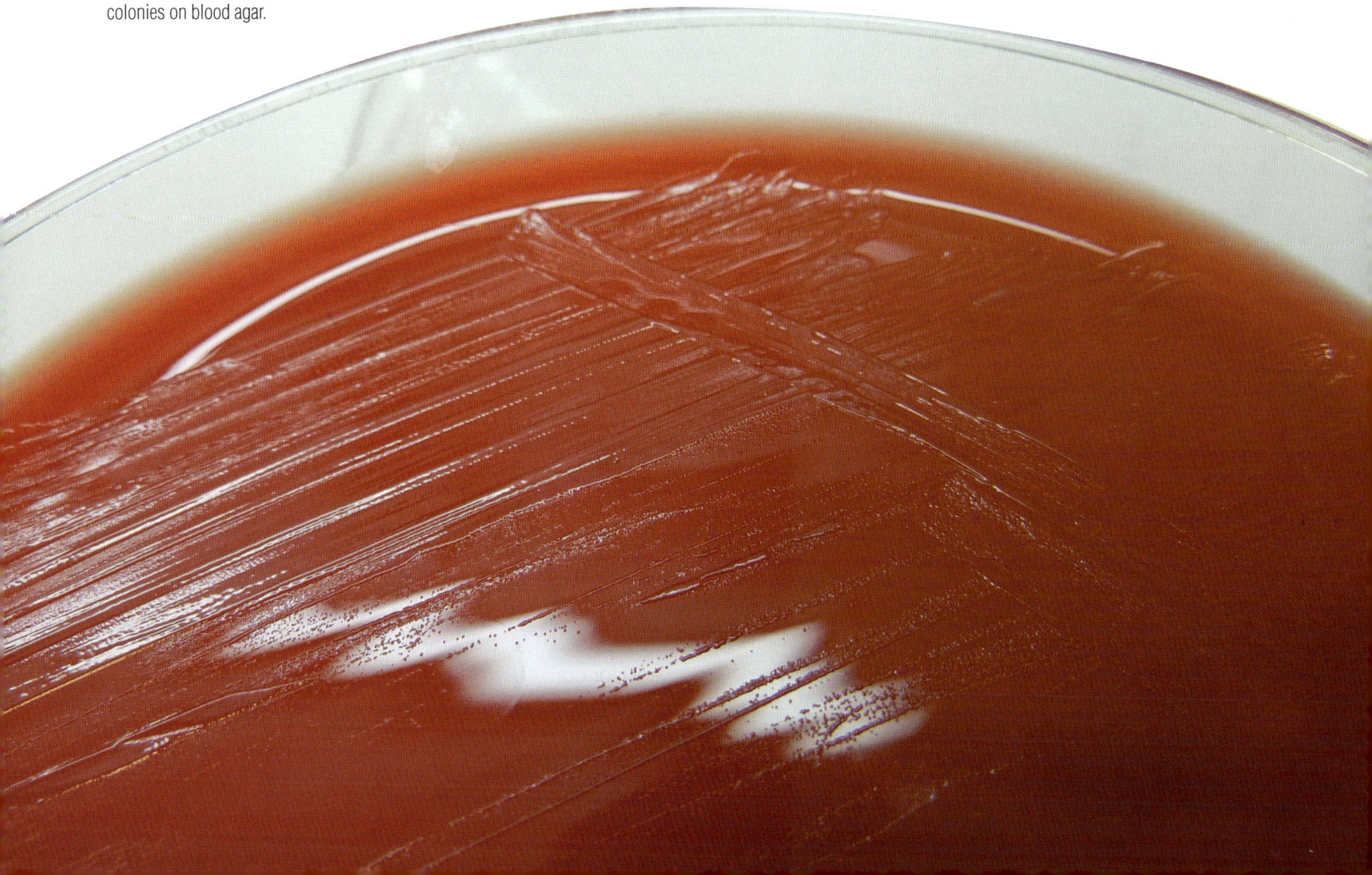

ORT has been shown to be highly sensitive to different chemical disinfectants. The most commonly used disinfectants are based on the antibacterial effects of different organic acids such as formic and glyoxylic acids, and on aldehydes that readily inactivate ORT *in vitro*. ORT was completely inactivated by a 0.5 % solution containing formic and glyoxylic acid and by a 0.5 % solution of an aldehyde-based product (20 % glutaraldehyde) after 15 minutes exposure time (Hafez and Schulze, 2003).

Several attempts to combat the infection using vaccines were carried out with different results. Vaccination trials with an inactivated vaccine in broilers, broiler breeders as well as in turkey flocks were carried out.

Vaccination of broiler breeders with an inactivated vaccine at 12th and 18th week of age also induces high antibody titers, which are passed to progenies and supply the offspring with a good protection against an ORT challenge for 14–30 days. The protection, however, decreases with increasing age of the progenies. On the other hand, investigating the effect of ORT vaccination of broiler breeders on antibody titers and performance of breeders and broilers revealed no differences in performance between vaccinated and unvaccinated breeders. However, a significantly lower mean mortality rate and higher mean production index in the broilers derived from vaccinated breeders could be observed (de Herdt et al., 2012).

In the field, vaccinations with autogenic inactivated oil-adjuvant vaccines were proven to be successful in reducing the outbreaks of ORT in turkeys and are widely used in some countries.

Using live vaccines at 1st day of age in broiler did not induce protection, while application of the vaccine at 7th or 14th days of age resulted in a good protection after experimental challenge. A temperature sensitive mutant of ORT also had some protective properties (Chin et al., 2013).

The importance of the serotype for vaccination is not well understood. It is generally assumed that protection after vaccination with inactivated vaccines is serotype specific, but it was shown that cross-protective immunity against different ORT serotypes can be induced by live vaccination.

References

CHIN RP, VAN EMPEL PCM AND HAFEZ HM. *Ornithobacterium rhinotracheale* infection. In: Diseases of Poultry, 13th edition, edited by DE Swayne, JR Glisson, LR McDougald, LK Nolan, DL Suarez and V Nair, eds. Iowa State Press, Ames, Iowa. 2013; pp. 828–834.

DE HERDT P, BROECKX M, VANKEIRSBILCK W, VAN DEN ABEELE G AND VAN GORP S. Improved broiler performance associated with *Ornithobacterium rhinotracheale* vaccination in breeders. *Avian Diseases*. 2012; 56(2): 365–368.

GORNATTI CHURRIA CD, MACHUCA MA, VIGO GB AND PETRUCCELLI MA. *Ornithobacterium rhinotracheale* infection in poultry: an updated review. *International Journal of Molecular Zoology*. 2012; 2(3): 23–38.

HAFEZ HM. Current status on the laboratory diagnosis of *Ornithobacterium rhinotracheale* "ORT" in poultry. *Berliner Münchener Tierärztliche Wochenschrift*. 1998; 111(4): 143–145.

HAFEZ HM AND SCHULZE D. Examinations on the efficacy of chemical disinfectants on *Ornithobacterium rhinotracheale* in vitro. *Archiv für Geflügelkunde*. 2003; 67: 153–156.

HAFEZ HM AND STING R. Investigations on different *Ornithobacterium rhinotracheale* "ORT" isolates. *Avian Diseases*. 1999; 43(1): 1–7.

HAFEZ HM AND VANDAMME P. Genus XXVI. *Ornithobacterium*. In: Bergey's manual of systematic bacteriology, 2nd edition, edited by NR Krieg, JT Staley, DR Brown, BP Hedlund, BJ Paster, NL Ward, W Ludwig and WB Whitman, eds. Springer, Williams & Wilkins, New York. 2011; pp. 250–314.

HAUCK R, CHIN RP AND SHIVAPRASAD HL. Retrospective study on the isolation of *Ornithobacterium rhinotracheale* from chickens and turkeys in central California: 294 cases (2000–12). *Avian Diseases*. 2015; 59(1): 130–137.

MARIEN M, DECOSTERE A, DUCHATEAU L, CHIERS K, FROYMAN R AND NAUWYNCK H. Efficacy of enrofloxacin, florfenicol and amoxicillin against *Ornithobacterium rhinotracheale* and *Escherichia coli* O2:K1 dual infection in turkeys following APV priming. *Veterinary Microbiology*. 2007; 121(1–2): 94–104.

MARIEN M, DECOSTERE A, MARTEL A, CHIERS K, FROYMAN R AND NAUWYNCK H. Synergy between avian pneumovirus and *Ornithobacterium rhinotracheale* in turkeys. *Avian Pathology*. 2005; 34(3): 204–211.

NUMEE S, HAUCK R AND HAFEZ HM. Influence of different storage media, temperatures and time duration on susceptibility of *Ornithobacterium rhinotracheale*. *Pakistan Veterinary Journal*. 2012; 32(3): 438–442.

VAN EMPEL PCM AND HAFEZ HM. *Ornithobacterium rhinotracheale*: a review. *Avian Pathology*. 1999; 28(3): 217–227.

6 *Riemerella anatipestifer* infection

Infections with *Riemerella anatipestifer* cause a septicaemic disease, which can manifest itself in the respiratory or gastrointestinal tract, as well as cause lesions in joints and central nervous signs. The disease can be acute or chronic, and has a worldwide distribution.

Young ducks followed by turkeys are most susceptible to infections.

Economic losses are due to increased mortality, bad feed conversion, decreased weight gain and high condemnation rates, as well as high medication cost.

Aetiology

R. anatipestifer is a rod-shaped and slightly curved, gram-negative, capsulated bacterium measuring 0.2–0.4 µm × 1.0–2.5 µm (Fig. 1). The cells are non-motile and do not form spores; they usually occur singly but can also form chains. *R. anatipestifer* is oxidase and catalase positive. It prefers high concentrations of CO_2 in the atmosphere.

After its first isolation from geese in 1904, it was renamed several times and placed into various genera including *Haemophilus*, *Pfeifferella* and *Pasteurella*. Today, *Riemerella* is recognized as a genus of its own within the

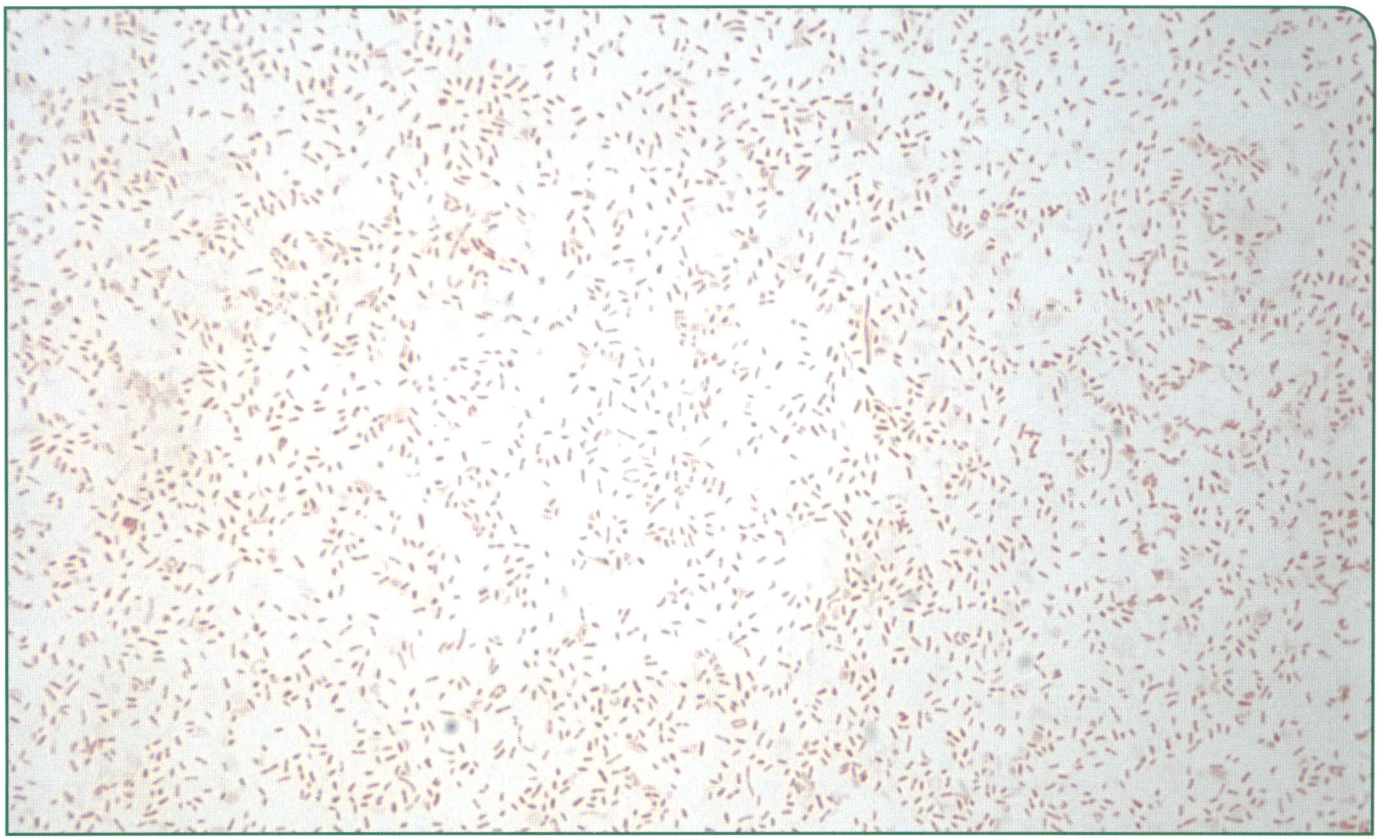

Figure 1. *Riemerella anatipestifer* cells. Gram stain. Image courtesy of Dr. Sarah Brüggemann-Schwarze (Institute for Poultry Diseases, Freie Universität Berlin).

Chapter co-authored by Dr. H.L. Shivaprasad (California Animal Health and Food Safety Laboratory System, Tulare branch).

family Flavobacteriaceae. This sets it clearly apart from *Pasteurella*, which are in another phylum, but reflects some similarity to *Ornithobacterium rhinotracheale*. In addition to *R. anatipestifer*, it contains the species *R. columbina* and *R. columbipharyngis*, which infect pigeons (Segers et al., 1993; Rubbenstroth et al., 2013a).

Besides ducks and turkeys, its host spectrum comprises other bird species including chickens, geese, pheasants, quail, and wild free-living waterfowl. It has also been isolated from pigs.

R. anatipestifer has a low tenacity but can survive up to 4 weeks in turkey litter.

Pathogenesis and transmission

Infection via inhalation is thought to be the most important route. However, under experimental conditions, infections by aerosol or injection into the abdominal air sac as well as oral infection do not fully reproduce the disease. Therefore, under field conditions, either co-infection with respiratory viruses such as avian metapneumovirus (aMPV) might be necessary for full development of the disease in turkeys (Rubbenstroth et al., 2009) or infection through small injuries of the skin might be more important. Mostly based on the seasonal occurrence, it has been suggested that mosquitoes can act as vectors (Ruiz and Sandhu, 2013).

After infection via the respiratory route, *R. anatipestifer* enters the blood by unknown mechanisms causing septicaemia and spreads throughout other organs. The bacterium has the ability to invade cells. During the last few years several potential virulence genes have been described. These include proteins involved in adhesion, iron acquisition and biofilm formation.

The bacterium is shed via the upper respiratory tract for up to 14 days after infection (Rubbenstroth et al., 2009); shedding in faeces occurs rarely.

Clinical signs

Clinical signs usually become apparent 2–5 days post-infection. Ducks between 1 and 8 weeks of age are highly susceptible. Diseased ducklings are depressed and lose weight. Mucous discharge is present in eyes and nares (Fig. 2), and birds have diarrhoea. Central nervous manifestations are common; birds show tremor of head and neck and lie on their back performing uncoordinated movements with their legs. Young ducks usually die 2 days after the onset of clinical signs. In older birds, the disease is rarer and takes a more protracted course in which birds can develop swollen joints.

Severity of the presentation of the disease depends on the infecting strain, co-infections with other respiratory pathogens and route of exposure. Depending on those factors, morbidity and mortality can be up close to 100 %, but also considerably less.

Turkeys are most susceptible between 5 and 15 weeks of age. Most common symptoms are respiratory distress, lameness and torticollis. Morbidity and mortality may be up to 60 %.

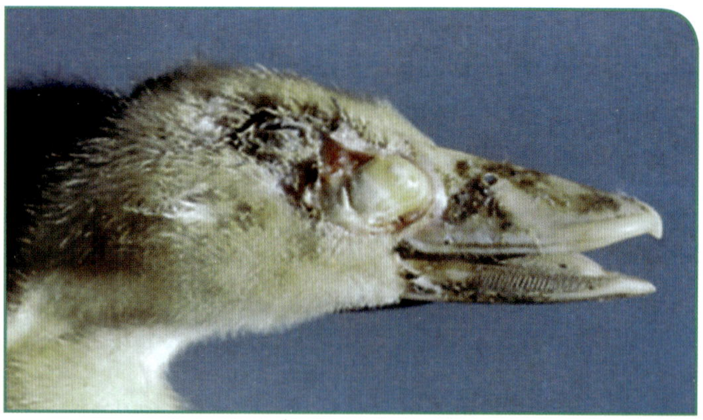

Figure 2. Nasal and ocular discharge and fibrinous exudate in the sinus of a duckling infected with *Riemerella anatipestifer*. Image courtesy of Clinic for Poultry (University of Veterinary Medicine Hannover).

Post mortem lesions

Gross lesions in ducks and turkeys are characterized by fibrinous polyserositis; pericarditis, perihepatitis and airsacculitis (Fig. 3) and fibrinous exudate in the air sacs. In laying ducks, the oviduct is often inflamed and filled with caseous material. Other localized, mostly fibrinous inflammations including dermatitis, arthritis, osteomyelitis, meningitis (Fig. 4) and focal pneumonia can be present. Additionally, the spleen may be swollen and mottled.

Microscopically, inflammations are characterized by fibrinous exudate containing mononuclear inflammatory cells and heterophils. Hepatocytes may show cloudy swelling and hydropic degeneration.

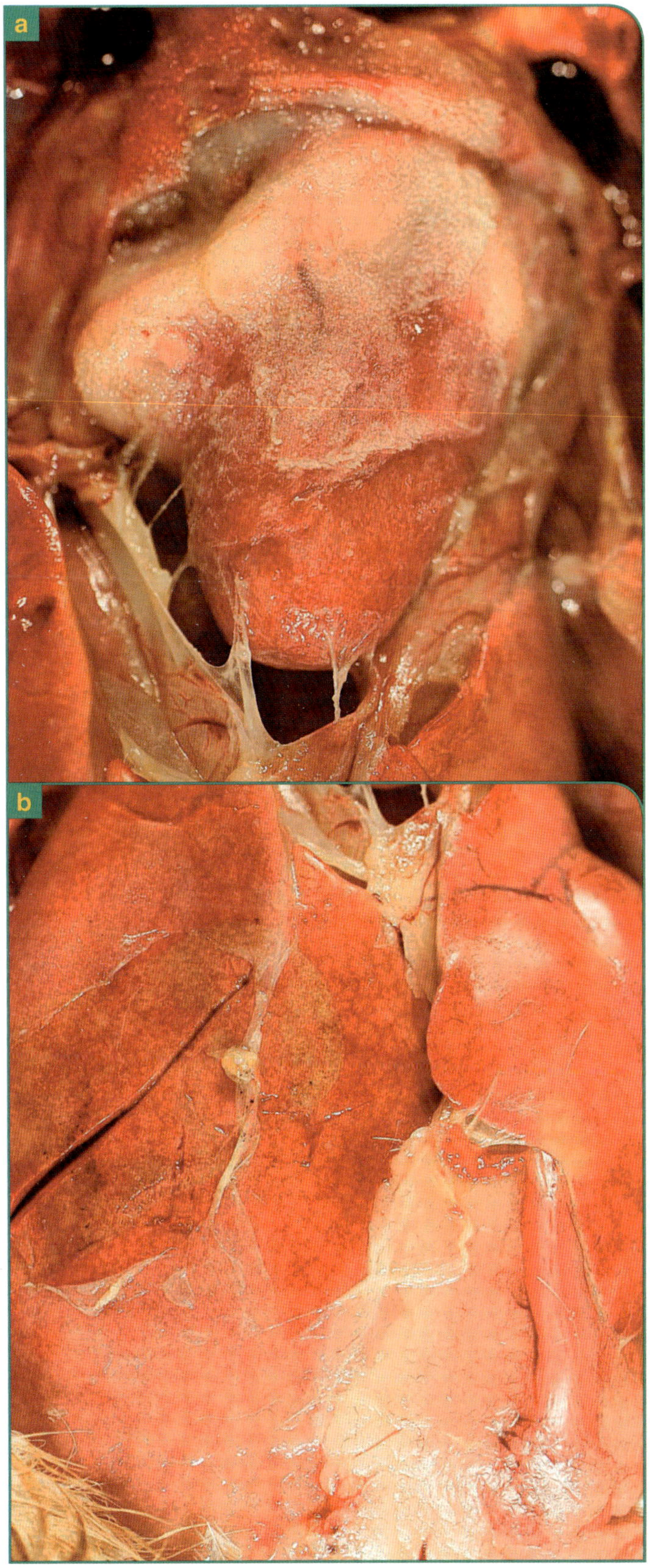

Figure 3. (a) Pericarditis and (b) perihepatitis in the sinus of a duckling infected with *Riemerella anatipestifer.* Image courtesy of Dr. H.L. Shivaprasad (California Animal Health and Food Safety Laboratory System, Tulare branch).

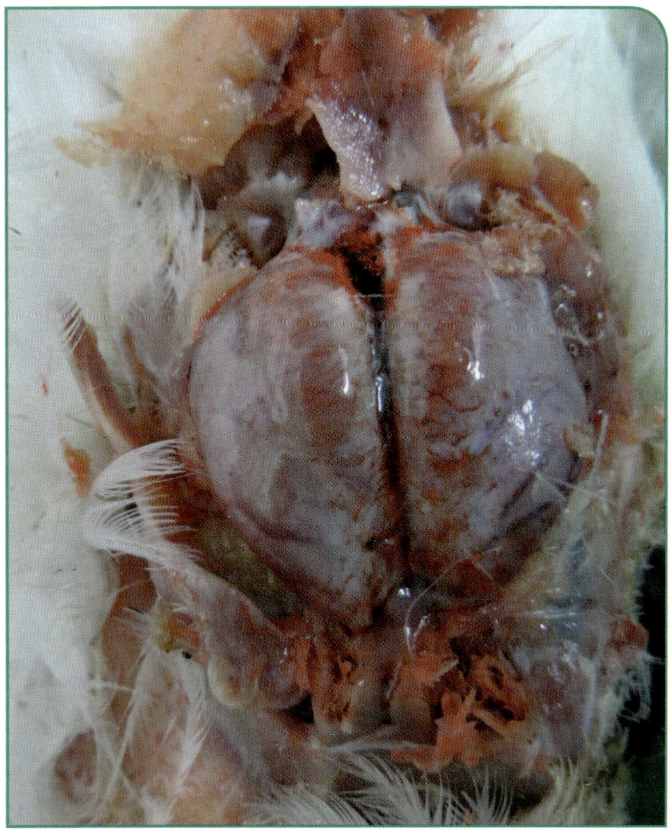

Figure 4. Meningitis in a goose after infection with *Riemerella anatipestifer.* Image courtesy of Dr. Erwin Sieverding (Praxis am Bergweg, Lohne).

Diagnostic procedures

Because other septicaemic diseases cause very similar symptoms and gross lesions, definitive diagnosis requires isolation and/or detection of *R. anatipestifer*.

The bacterium can be isolated relatively easy during the acute stage of the disease from various organs including liver, lung, spleen, heart, blood, kidney and brain.

Since the bacterium dies within few days at room temperature, shipping samples will negatively affect chances of isolation. Blood agar, chocolate agar, trypticase soy agar or other media containing blood or serum are suitable, but *R. anatipestifer* does not grow on MacConkey agar. Since most *R. anatipestifer* isolates are resistant to gentamicin, it has been suggested to add 5 mg/l gentamicin to plate media to suppress growth of other bacteria. Plates should be incubated for 24–48 hours at 35–38 °C. The atmosphere should be microaerophilic containing 5–10 % CO_2. Incubation under aerobic as well as anaerobic conditions will give suboptimal results. Colonies are smooth, non-pigmented or grayish-white to beige and non-haemolytic. They are usually transparent and 1–2 µm in diameter, but some strains show slimy growth (Fig. 5).

Identification of *R. anatipestifer* by its biochemical properties can be difficult, since many reactions are not consistent. *R. anatipestifer* is typically proteolytic, but does not ferment carbohydrates. Variable reactions include indole reaction as well as urease and gelatinase activity. Depending on the micro-test kit used, some enzyme reactions give variable results: β-glucosidase, α-galactosidase and lipase activity are positive in the API ID32E and negative in the API ZYM system, while N-acetyl-β-glucosaminidase are negative in API ZYM and API ID32E, but positive in LRA-ZYM-Oxidase (Hinz et al., 1998).

PCR can be used for detection of bacterial DNA directly in organ material as well as for identification of isolates (Tsai et al., 2005; Rubbenstroth et al., 2013b).

Typing of isolates can be done by plate agglutination, tube agglutination or agar gel precipitation assay. To date, at least 21 different serotypes have been identified by slide and tube agglutination tests (Loh et al., 1992; Pathanasophon et al., 1994). Serotypes seem not to be related with hosts or virulence. Reference sera for serotyping are commercially available in Europe, but several typing systems designating serotypes with numbers or letters have been used in the past and are still in use (Rubbenstroth et al., 2013b; Ruiz and Sandhu, 2013). This makes comparing results between laboratories and publications difficult and

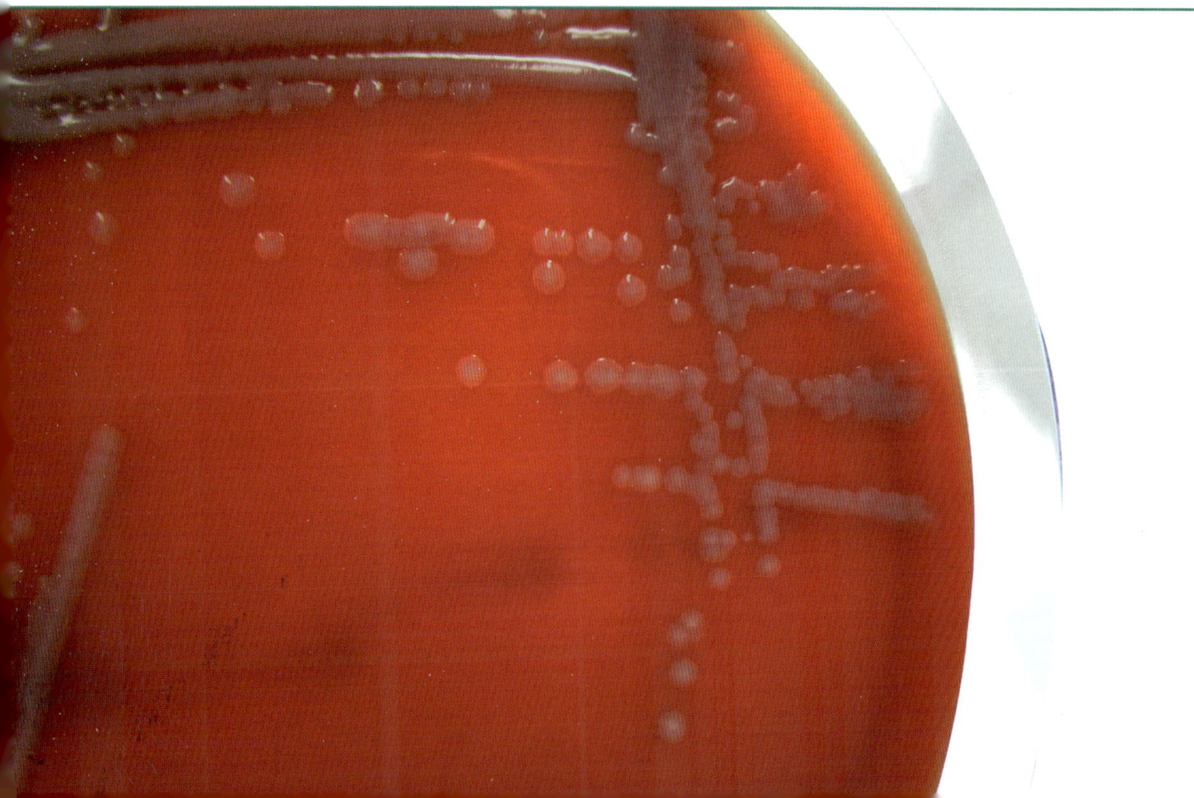

Figure 5. *Riemerella anatipestifer* colonies on blood agar. Image courtesy of Dr. Sarah Brüggemann-Schwarze (Institute for Poultry Diseases, Freie Universität Berlin).

confusing. Additionally, cross-reactions between various reference sera occur.

Molecular biological methods for typing that have been used for epidemiological studies include sequencing of the 16s rRNA gene, whole genome restriction enzyme analysis followed by pulsed-field gel electrophoresis (PFGE) or repetitive-sequence PCR.

Agglutination as well as an ELISA assay for detection of antibodies against *R. anatipestifer* have been described. However, they are not commercially available and their usefulness in routine diagnostic is limited due to the short incubation period of the disease.

Treatment

Flocks with riemerellosis should be treated with antibiotics in drinking water or via feed to reduce morbidity and mortality. However, selection of suitable antibiotics is difficult, especially for ducks, for which only very few antibiotics are registered. In addition, sensitivity and resistance of *R. anatipestifer* isolates vary considerably, so sensitivity test should be carried out on a routine base in order to determine the current and local situation. Several methods including disk diffusion and microdilution using various media have been described and used for antibacterial susceptibility testing of *R. anatipestifer*. However, no standard methods and breakpoints have been established. In recent years, several resistance genes of *R. anatipestifer* have been described, which in the future might be used for assays to predict resistance.

Generally, *R. anatipestifer* is considered to be resistant against the polypeptide antibiotics polymyxin B and colistin as well as against aminoglycoside antibiotics kanamycin and gentamicin. Information regarding the effectiveness of tetracyclines is inconsistent. While their role in therapy of riemerellosis has been described "of little value", and resistance genes against tetracyclines seem to be common, *in vitro* testing indicated low levels of resistance (Zhong et al., 2009; Ruiz and Sandhu, 2013).

Antibiotics that can be considered to treat infections with *R. anatipestifer* include sulphonamides with or without pyrimidine potentiator, aminopenicillins and other beta-lactams, macrolides, lincomycin alone or lincomycin-spectinomycin and enrofloxacin. Treatment should continue for at least 3 days.

Control

Routine biosecurity measures can prevent the introduction of *R. anatipestifer* and other pathogens that might predispose to an infection with *R. anatipestifer* or aggravate the morbidity, mortality and severity of symptoms into flocks. Thorough cleaning and disinfection of houses between flocks will decrease infection pressure with those pathogens. Other predisposing factors that can be minimized are bad air quality, high stocking densities or extreme temperatures.

Specific prevention can be achieved by vaccination. Since no vaccine is commercially available, autogenous vaccines have to be used.

The protection offered by inactivated whole-cell or bacterin vaccines is almost completely serotype specific and vaccination with them does not confer adequate protection against other serotypes. For that reason, a vaccine should contain several serotypes, if technically and legally possible. Using formalin-inactivated bacterins with aluminum hydroxide gel as adjuvant provides protection only for 2 weeks, while oil-emulsion adjuvant provides a longer protection, which lasts until slaughter of fattening ducks at 42 days of age after a single vaccination (Liu et al., 2013). During the first days of life, ducklings can also be protected by maternal antibodies induced by vaccination of the breeder flock. Naturally avirulent strains have been successfully used as live vaccine (Sandhu, 1991). Published research into vaccination of turkeys against *R. anatipestifer* is lacking.

References

Hinz KH, Ryll M, Kohler B and Glünder G. Phenotypic characteristics of *Riemerella anatipestifer* and similar microorganisms from various hosts. *Avian Pathology*. 1998; 27, 33–42.

Liu H, Wang X, Ding C, Han X, Cheng A, Wang S and Yu S. Development and evaluation of a trivalent *Riemerella anatipestifer*-inactivated vaccine. *Clinical and Vaccine Immunology*. 2013; 20, 691–697.

Loh H, Teo TP and Tan HC. Serotypes of "*Pasteurella*" *anatipestifer* isolates from ducks in Singapore: a proposal of new serotypes. *Avian Pathology*. 1992; 21, 453–459.

Pathanasophon P, Tanticharoenyos T and Sawada T. Physiological characteristics, antimicrobial susceptibility and serotypes of *Pasteurella anatipestifer* isolated from ducks in Thailand. *Veterinary Microbiolo*gy. 1994; 39, 179–185.

Rubbenstroth D, Ryll M, Behr K-P and Rautenschlein S. Pathogenesis of *Riemerella anatipestifer* in turkeys after experimental mono-infection via respiratory routes or dual infection together with the avian metapneumovirus. *Avian Pathology*. 2009; 38, 497–507.

Rubbenstroth D, Ryll M, Hotzel H, Christensen H, Knobloch JK-M, Rautenschlein S and Bisgaard M. Description of *Riemerella columbipharyngis* sp. nov., isolated from the pharynx of healthy domestic pigeons (Columba livia f. domestica), and emended descriptions of the genus *Riemerella*, *Riemerella anatipestifer* and *Riemerella columbina*. *International Journal of Systematic and Evolutionary Microbiology*. 2013a; 63, 280–287.

Rubbenstroth D, Ryll M, Knobloch JK-M, Köhler B and Rautenschlein S. Evaluation of different diagnostic tools for the detection and identification of *Riemerella anatipestifer*. *Avian Pathology*. 2013b; 42, 17–26.

Ruiz JA and Sandhu TS. Riemerella anatipestifer infection. In: Diseases of Poultry, DE Swayne, JR Glisson, LR McDougald, LK Nolan, DL Suarez and V Nair, eds. Ames, Iowa: Wiley-Blackwell. 2013; pp. 823–828.

Sandhu TS. Immunogenicity and safety of a live *Pasteurella anatipestifer* vaccine in White Pekin ducklings: Laboratory and field trials. *Avian Pathology*. 1991; 20, 423–432.

Segers P, Mannheim W, Vancanneyt M, De Brandt K, Hinz KH, Kersters K and Vandamme P. *Riemerella anatipestifer* gen. nov., comb. nov., the causative agent of septicemia anserum exsudativa, and its phylogenetic affiliation within the Flavobacterium-Cytophaga rRNA homology group. *International Journal of Systematic Bacteriology*. 1993; 43, 768–776.

Tsai H-J, Liu Y-T, Tseng C-S and Pan M-J. Genetic variation of the ompA and 16S rRNA genes of *Riemerella anatipestifer*. *Avian Pathology*. 2005; 34, 55–64.

Zhong CY, Cheng AC, Wang MS, Zhu DK, Luo QH, De Zhong C, Li L and Duan Z. Antibiotic susceptibility of *Riemerella anatipestifer* field isolates. *Avian Diseases*. 2009; 53, 601–607.

7 Infectious coryza

Infectious coryza of chickens is caused by infection with *Avibacterium paragallinarum*, which was previously known as *Haemophilus paragallinarum*, and should not be confused with turkey coryza, which is caused by *Bordetella* spp. As its name suggests, it is primarily a catarrhal inflammation of the mucous membranes of the upper respiratory tract. However, even without complicating infections, it can cause poor productivity of infected birds and, in rare cases, lead to high condemnation rates due to airsacculitis, both causing economic losses. The disease is ubiquitous in intensive production and village poultry.

Aetiology

Av. paragallinarum is a gram-negative, rod-shaped, non-motile, and oxidase-positive bacterium. Some strains are capsulated. The rods are short, measuring between 1–3 µm in length and 0.4–0.8 µm in width. In older cultures, bacterial cells will lose their form.

The genus *Avibacterium*, with its five species, belongs to the family Pasteurellaceae. The current taxonomy is based on the 16s rRNA sequences. The species *Av. paragallinarum* comprises the former distinct species *Pasteurella gallinarum*, *P. avium*, *P. volantium* and *H. paragallinarum* (Blackall et al., 2005). *H. paragallinarum* in turn also comprised the apocryphal species *H. gallinarum*. *H. gallinarum* is supposed to differ from *H. paragallinarum* in that it requires both haemin (X-factor) and nicotinamide adenine dinucleotide (NAD, V-factor) for growth, while *H. paragallinarum* requires no haemin and sometimes no NAD; there has been no recent description of *Av. paragallinarum* isolates requiring haemin for growth.

It should be explicitly noted that the presently recognized species *Av. gallinarum* is not identical with the historical species *H. gallinarum*.

Avibacterium species other than *Av. paragallinarum* are considered to be avirulent and might be combined into fewer species in the future (Bisgaard et al., 2012).

Three serogroups designated A, B and C are distinguished by haemagglutination inhibition (HI) test using washed bacterial cells and glutaraldehyde-fixed chicken erythrocytes. This test is superior to the historically used plate agglutination test. Using thiocyanate-treated and sonicated cells instead of whole cells as antigen increases the discriminatory power of the test. With this method, currently nine serovars are recognized within the serogroups. The serovars are designated A-1, A-2, A-3, A-4, B-1, C-1, C-2, C-3 and C-4 (Blackall et al., 1990).

Av. paragallinarum is not stable in the environment. It remains infectious only for few days in exudate outside the host.

Pathogenesis and transmission

Infection takes place by the respiratory route.

Due to the low tenacity of *Av. paragallinarum*, clinically infected chickens and/or carriers are the main reservoir and the most important vectors; chickens can remain infected and continue to shed the bacterium from the upper respiratory tract after overcoming disease.

Thus, multiple-age farms are at special risk. The bacterium can spread between birds through aerosols or via drinking water contaminated with nasal discharge from diseased birds.

Wild birds do not seem to play a role as vectors since reports of isolation of *Av. paragallinarum* from other bird species are regarded as not sufficiently substantiated. Turkeys, pigeons, sparrows, ducks and crows were refractory to experimental infection, making it unlikely that other bird species are important hosts. There is no vertical transmission (Blackall and Soriano-Vargas, 2013).

Typically, the infection remains restricted to the upper respiratory tract. In some cases, however, the bacteria spread to the lungs and the air sacs even without other respiratory pathogens present. Spread to the lower respiratory tract might be associated with NAD-independence (Horner et al., 1995).

Virulence of isolates is dependent on the ability of the strains to adhere to the respiratory epithelium, which is mediated by the capsule as well as by the haemagglutination antigen. One investigation showed that strains lacking a capsule did not attach to the cilia and were avirulent. The capsule is also thought to protect the bacterial cells against the non-specific immune response of the host. Furthermore, like the capsule, the haemagglutinating antigen is involved in attachment (Sawata et al., 1985). On the other hand, a more recent investigation showed that a deletion mutant not producing a capsule had increased haemagglutination and adhesion activities, but decreased the virulence in chickens (Tu et al., 2014).

Proteins involved in iron acquisition have been described and are considered virulence factors. Furthermore, *Av. paragallinarum* produces several toxins, which are probably released in vesicles. Recent studies identified several toxins including a serine-protease-RTX toxin and a cytolethal distending toxin (Küng and Frey, 2013; Chen et al., 2014).

Infection with *Av. paragallinarum* also seems to attract large numbers of mast cells that mediate the inflammation causing damage.

Cases in which *Av. paragallinarum* spread throughout the body in the presence of other pathogens have been reported (Sandoval et al., 1994). It is unclear if septicaemia or bacteraemia occurred in these cases and if any special virulence factors of the causative strains or only the concurrent infections were responsible for this atypical behaviour.

Clinical signs

Clinical signs develop after a relatively short incubation period of 1 to 3 days and, in cases not complicated by the presence of other pathogens, will subside after 2 to 3 weeks.

While chickens of all ages develop the disease after infection, severity of the disease tends to increase with age, being active laying hens the most susceptible.

Apart from the age of chickens, severity of signs depends on co-infection with other respiratory pathogens and on environmental conditions. Depending on those factors, morbidities of up to 50 %, mortalities of up to 20 % and drops in egg production of up to 40 % have been described. Drops in egg production are probably mainly caused by decreased water consumption, while decreased feed consumption will lead to impaired growth rates.

Clinical signs are typical for infections of the upper respiratory tract. They are dominated by serous to mucoid nasal discharge and conjunctivitis (Figs. 1 and 2). In more complicated cases, head and wattles may be swollen as in swollen head syndrome (Fig. 3). Respiratory sounds can be audible if the lower respiratory tract is infected.

Post mortem lesions

In line with pathogenesis and clinical signs, pathological lesions usually only consist of an acute catarrhal inflammation of the upper respiratory tract, i.e. nasal mucosa, sinuses (Fig. 4), conjunctivae and trachea. The mucosae are reddened and covered by mucopurulent exudate. Microscopically, the mucous membranes are hyperaemic and oedematous with infiltration of heterophils and mast cells, while the epithelial cells are swollen and have lost their cilia. Oedematous swelling of the facial subcutaneous tissue and of the wattles can occur. If the lower respiratory tract is involved, catarrhal bronchopneumonia characterized by consolidated and congested lungs and cell debris in the lumen of the bronchi as well as catarrhal airsacculitis are present.

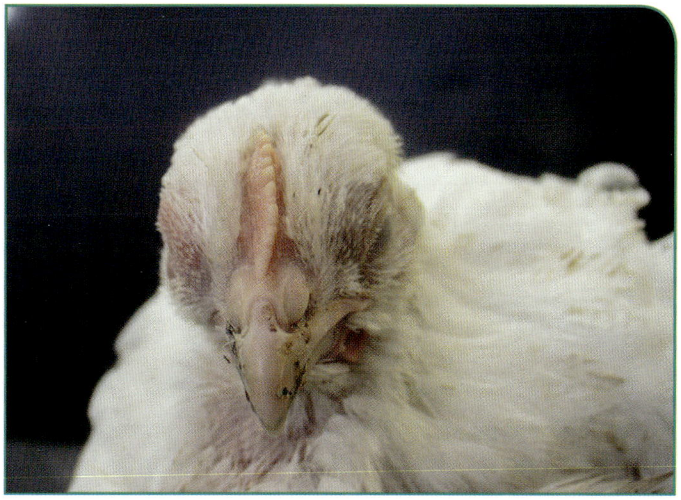

Figure 1. Young chicken with infectious coryza. Note respiratory exudate on the beak.

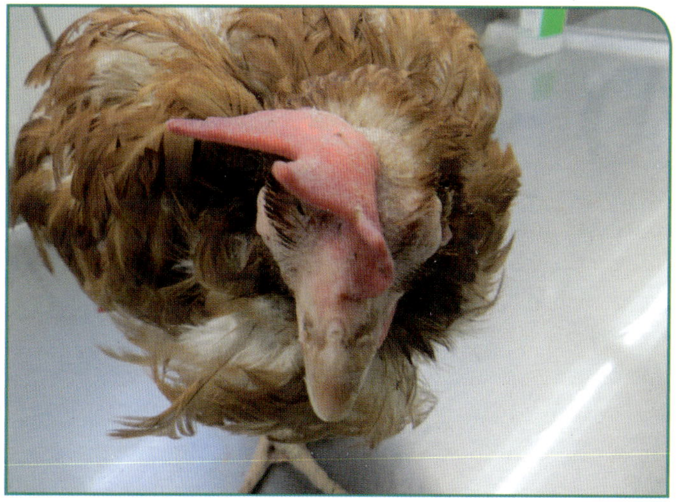

Figure 2. Laying hen with infectious coryza. Note respiratory exudate on the beak. Image courtesy of Dr. Erwin Sieverding (Praxis am Bergweg, Lohne).

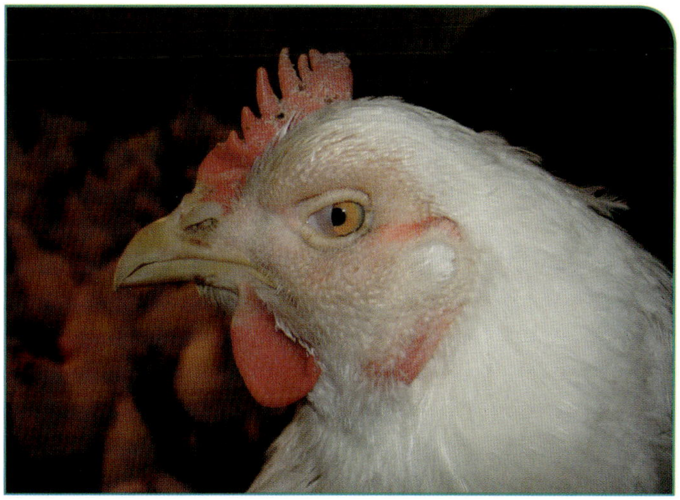

Figure 3. Laying hen with infectious coryza showing swollen eyelids due to conjunctivitis and facial oedema.

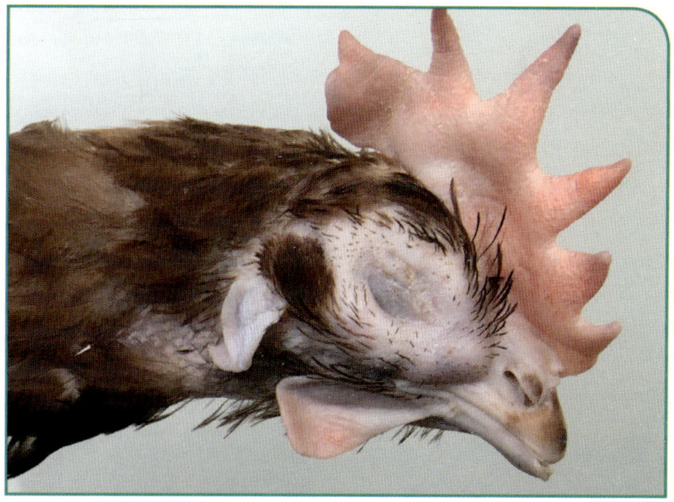

Figure 4. Laying hen with infectious coryza showing facial oedema and sinusitis. Image courtesy of Dr. Simone Stoute and Dr. Manuela Crispo (California Animal Health and Food Safety Laboratory System, Turlock branch).

Diagnostic procedures

After presumptive diagnosis based on clinical signs and lesions, definitive diagnosis can be made by isolation or detection of *Av. paragallinarum*. Preferred samples are swabs taken from inflamed sinuses; tracheal swabs can also be suitable.

> **Considering that *Av. paragallinarum* can be challenging to isolate and that, due to its fragile nature, may not survive when shipping samples, detection by PCR might be the most reliable method.**

A thoroughly validated PCR assay suitable for direct investigation of samples has been described, and is widely used (Chen et al., 1998).

Most common media for isolation are blood agar or brain heart infusion (BHI) agar. Most strains of *Av. paragallinarum* require the addition of NADH (1.56–25 µg/ml) or NAD$^+$ (20–100 µg/ml) to the medium. Alternatively, chocolate agar can be used or NAD can be substituted by a feeder bacterium. For this purpose, an NAD-producing *Staphylococcus* sp. strain, most commonly *S. epidermidis* or *S. hyicus*, is cross-streaked on the plate after plating of the diagnostic sample. Additionally, *Av. paragallinarum* requires an increased sodium chloride concentration between 1 % and 1.5 % for growth, and some strains require the addition of serum to BHI. Chicken, bovine and equine sera in concentrations up to 10 % have been used for that purpose. Plates should be incubated at 37 °C under microaerophilic or anaerobic conditions, often in an atmosphere containing 5 % CO_2.

Colonies are up to 0.3 mm in diameter and dewdrop-like (Fig. 5). If a feeder strain is used, NAD-dependent *Av. paragallinarum* will only grow close to the feeder colonies. Biochemical identification tests for identification and differentiation from other, non-pathogenic *Avibacterium* spp. or similar bacteria include a positive catalase test, no acid production from L-arabinose, D-mannitol and D-sorbitol and acid production from D-galactose, maltose and trehalose. More complete characteristics and practical aspects for biochemical characterization have been described by Blackall and Soriano-Vargas (2013).

As described above, HI test is the standard test for serotyping isolates. Apart from the original plate agglutination test, other methods described are agar gel precipitation test and the use of monoclonal antibodies. A multiplex PCR designed to detect serotypes did not yield satisfying results (Morales-Erasto et al., 2014). For epidemiological studies, molecular typing techniques like ribotyping, ERIC-PCR and multilocus sequence typing (MLST) have been used.

Antibodies can be detected by HI test, by blocking ELISA, which is serotype specific for serogroups A and C, but not available to detect antibodies against serogroup B, and by ELISA using recombinant antigen. Due to the acute nature of the disease, it is most useful to monitor antibody levels after vaccination. Chickens with an antibody titer of 1:5 in the HI or 0.3 in the ELISA can be considered protected (Sawata et al., 1982; Sakamoto et al., 2012).

Treatment

Antibiotic therapy of infectious coryza should be considered since it can improve clinical signs. However, it will not clear the birds from the infection, so clinical signs can reoccur after the end of the therapy and chickens will continue to shed the bacteria.

Sulfonamides, erythromycin and oxytetracycline have been recommended but, while development of antibiotic resistance has been described, there are virtually no recent publications about the current resistance situation.

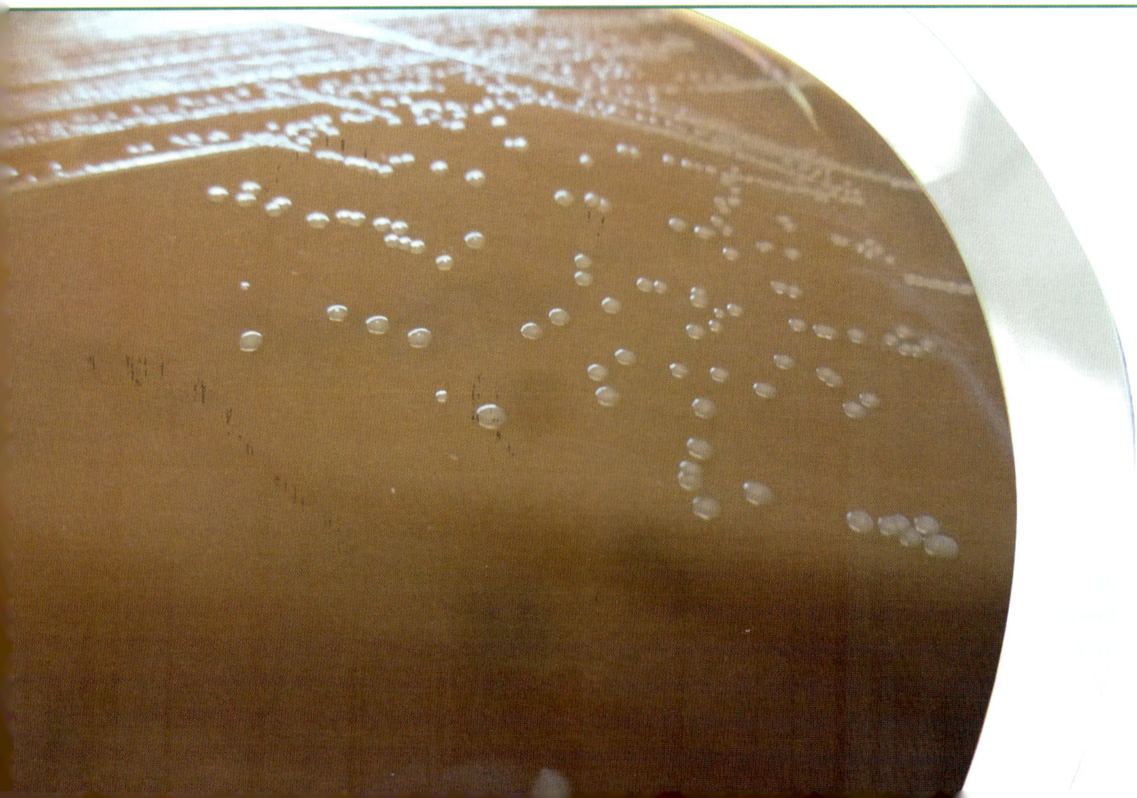

Figure 5. *Avibacterium paragallinarum* colonies on chocolate agar. Image courtesy of Dr. Kristin Mühldorfer (Leibniz-Institut für Zoo- und Wildtierforschung, Berlin).

Control

When devising preventive measures against infectious coryza, it should be kept in mind that infected chickens are the main vectors and the bacterium can be spread by the airborne route.

Breaking this infectious cycle between different flocks on a farm is the most important.

Flocks should be strictly separated if they are not the same age. Houses and equipment should be thoroughly cleaned and disinfected. A waiting time of 2 to 3 weeks before restocking will help to eliminate the bacterium. Obviously, houses should only be restocked with birds that never underwent an infection with *Av. paragallinarum*.

Inactivated whole-cell vaccines against infectious coryza are commercially available in many countries. Active laying hens, which are most susceptible to infectious coryza, should be vaccinated between 10 weeks of age and the onset of lay in order to be protected. A booster vaccination after 4 weeks will improve the protection, which will last for months.

The protection conferred by vaccination is serogroup specific, but vaccines containing two serogroups can protect against disease after infection with an isolate belonging to the third serogroup. However, this does not apply universally and most, if not all, commercial vaccines contain all three serogroups. Cross-protection between different serovars within one serogroup seems to be common, but can only be partial. This is applied especially for serogroup B, which comprises only serovar B-1. Thus, in case of repeated vaccination failure, the use of autogenous vaccines can be considered.

In contrast, immunity after natural infection is not serogroup specific. However, attempts to develop attenuated vaccines seem to be totally lacking.

References

Bisgaard M, Nørskov-Lauritsen N, de Wit SJ, Hess C and Christensen H. Multilocus sequence phylogenetic analysis of *Avibacterium. Microbiology.* 2012; 158, 993–1004.

Blackall PJ and Soriano-Vargas E. Infectious coryza and related bacterial infections. In: Diseases of Poultry, DE Swayne, JR Glisson, LR McDougald, LK Nolan, DL Suarez and V Nair, eds. Ames, Iowa: Wiley-Blackwell. 2013; pp. 859–873.

Blackall PJ, Eaves LE and Rogers DG. Proposal of a new serovar and altered nomenclature for *Haemophilus paragallinarum* in the Kume hemagglutinin scheme. *Journal of Clinical Microbiology.* 1990; 28, 1185–1187.

Blackall PJ, Christensen H, Beckenham T, Blackall LL and Bisgaard M. Reclassification of *Pasteurella gallinarum*, [*Haemophilus*] *paragallinarum*, *Pasteurella avium* and *Pasteurella volantium* as *Avibacterium gallinarum* gen. nov., comb. nov., *Avibacterium paragallinarum* comb. nov., *Avibacterium avium* comb. nov. and *Avibacterium volantium* comb. nov. *International Journal of Systematic and Evolutionary Microbiology.* 2005; 55, 353–362.

Chen X, Song C, Gong Y and Blackall PJ. Further studies on the use of a polymerase chain reaction test for the diagnosis of infectious coryza. *Avian Pathology.* 1998; 27, 618–624.

Chen Y-C, Tan D-H, Shien J-H, Hsieh M-K, Yen T-Y and Chang P-C. Identification and functional analysis of the cytolethal distending toxin gene from *Avibacterium paragallinarum. Avian Pathology.* 2014; 43, 43–50.

Horner RF, Bishop GC, Jarvis CJ and Coetzer THT. NAD (V-factor) - independent and typical *Haemophilus paragallinarum* infection in commercial chickens: A five year field study. *Avian Pathology.* 1995; 24, 453–463.

Küng E and Frey J. AvxA, a composite serine-protease-RTX toxin of *Avibacterium paragallinarum. Veterinary Microbiology.* 2013; 163, 290–298.

Morales-Erasto V, Posadas-Quintana J de J, Fernández-Díaz M, Saravia LE, Martínez-Castañeda JS, Blackall PJ and Soriano-Vargas E. An evaluation of serotyping of *Avibacterium paragallinarum* by use of a multiplex polymerase chain reaction. *Journal of Veterinary Diagnostic Investigation.* 2014; 26, 272–276.

Sakamoto R, Sakai T, Ushijima T, Imamura T, Kino Y, Honda T and Sakaguchi M. Development of an enzyme-linked immunosorbent assay for the measurement of antibodies against infectious coryza vaccine. *Avian Diseases.* 2012; 56, 65–72.

Sandoval VE, Terzolo HR and Blackall PJ. Complicated infectious coryza outbreaks in Argentina. *Avian Diseases.* 1994; 38, 672–678.

Sawata A, Kume K and Nakase Y. Hemagglutinin of *Haemophilus-paragallinarum* serotype-2 organisms - occurrence and immunological properties of hemagglutinin. *American Journal of Veterinary Research.* 1982; 43, 1311–1314.

Sawata A, Nakai T, Kume K, Yoshikawa H and Yoshikawa T. Intranasal inoculation of chickens with encapsulated or non-encapsulated variants of *Haemophilus paragallinarum*: electron microscopic evaluation of the nasal mucosa. *American Journal of Veterinary Research.* 1985; 46, 2346–2353.

Tu T-Y, Hsieh M-K, Tan D-H, Ou S-C, Shien J-H, Yen T-Y and Chang P-C. Loss of the capsule increases the adherence activity but decreases the virulence of *Avibacterium paragallinarum. Avian Diseases.* 2014; 59, 87–93.

8 Mycoplasmosis

Infections with *Mycoplasma* spp. are of great economic importance for commercial poultry. Mostly infection with *Mycoplasma* spp. does not cause clinical disease, but they predispose their hosts for infection with other pathogens. Alone or together with these pathogens, they are responsible for drop of egg production, poor feed conversion, decreased growth rates, high condemnation rates, increased medication costs and impaired reproductive performance. *Mycoplasma* spp. are nearly ubiquitous and difficult to control; great efforts have been made and are still made to obtain mycoplasma-free flocks by cleaning the production chain from the top. For poultry, *M. gallisepticum* (MG), *M. synoviae* (MS), *M. meleagridis* (MM) and *M. iowae* (MI) are the most relevant species. They cause disease of the respiratory tract and/or the musculoskeletal system. MG infections are often referred to as chronic respiratory disease (CRD), a term which also denotes infections with *Escherichia coli*. MS can cause inflammation of the air sacs, synovitis in the joints and tendovaginitis or drop of eggshell quality. Vertical infections with MM and MI can be responsible for airsacculitis and bone deformations.

Aetiology

Mycoplasmas are among the smallest self-replicating bacteria and they are the smallest bacteria that are not obligatory intracellular. Their coccoid to pleomorphic cells measure about 0.2–0.5 µm in diameter.

Their most distinct characteristic is the lack of a cell wall, being surrounded only by a cell membrane.

Due to that, mycoplasmas stain only weakly gram-negative but well with Giemsa. Their genome can be as small as 600 kbp, which is only double the size of the largest viruses.

Based on their lack of a cell wall, the genus *Mycoplasma* is grouped into the class Mollicutes. The genus comprises far more than 100 species and several candidate species. In general, *Mycoplasma* spp. have a narrow host spectrum, infecting only few species or even only a single one. Mycoplasmas have been found in most mammals and birds, and frequently yet undescribed *Mycoplasma* spp. are isolated from various hosts or their DNA is detected using PCR. More than 20 species that can infect avian hosts are officially acknowledged and more have been described, including the four pathogenic species mentioned above. Other species such as *M. imitans* can cause diseases in ducks and geese.

Because they lack a cell wall, mycoplasmas have a low tenacity. They survive for less than 1 week in the environment, and are easily inactivated by common disinfectants.

Pathogenesis and transmission

Birds get infected with mycoplasmas either vertically or horizontally via the respiratory route.

Once a bird is infected, it can remain a carrier of mycoplasma for life and continue to shed the bacteria. Consequently, infected birds, including wild birds, are the main reservoir.

Gallinaceous birds including chickens, turkeys, pheasants, quail and peafowl are the most important hosts of MG, but it has also been frequently isolated from ducks, geese and songbirds. In finches, MG causes a fatal disease. Additionally, there are reports about isolation of MG from exotic birds like Amazon parrots and flamingos, indicating a broader host range.

The host spectrum of MS comprises ducks, geese, pigeons, budgerigars and sparrows besides various gallinaceous birds. MM has been detected in quail, peafowl, pigeons and falcons, while chickens are refractory to infection. MI infects chickens, turkeys and geese, and has also been isolated from wild and exotic birds.

Horizontal spread of MG and MS occurs very efficiently by direct contact in aerosols or droplets, and in spite of the low tenacity, fomites play an important role.

In a noteworthy experiment, Christensen et al. (1994) showed that at least some MG isolates can survive inside the human nose for up to 1 day and on human hair for up to 3 days. On feathers MG stayed infective for up to 4 days and on inorganic material for up to 2 days. MM can spread in a similar way, but infection via the respiratory route is of limited importance since it will not cause disease. Horizontal spread of MI is very slow and not considered to be relevant. All mycoplasmas can cause venereal infections.

After respiratory infection, MG and MS colonize the surface of the respiratory mucosa and spread along those to the lower respiratory tract and within the air sacs throughout the body. Ovaries are thought to get infected due to their proximity to the air sacs. In contrast, MM will rarely and only in younger birds spread to the ovaries or other organs after respiratory infection (Raviv and Ley, 2013).

MG has the ability to enter cells and can also cause bacteraemia in some cases, and encephalitis due to MG probably following bacteraemia has been reported (Roberts and McDaniel, 1967; Wyrzykowski et al., 2013).

It is unclear how MS reaches synovial structures. Under experimental conditions, parenteral infection like footpad inoculation or *in ovo* infection will result more often in synovitis than respiratory infection, showing that the route of infection is important. On the other hand, some MS strains are more likely to cause either respiratory disease or tendosynovitis, indicating that virulence factors present in some strains contribute to the development of systemic infections (Kleven et al., 1975).

Vertical transmission of mycoplasmas can occur at high rates.

During the peak shedding phase, approximately 3 to 6 weeks after infection with MG or MS, up to 50 % of all hatching eggs in a breeder flock can be contaminated; after that, the transmission rate decreases to 5 % or below (Roberts and McDaniel, 1967; Sasipreeyajan et al., 1987). However, even if only very few chicks are vertically infected at hatch, these will quickly horizontally infect the other birds of the same hatch and/or the flock during rearing. Infections with MG and/or MS alone will usually not cause clinical disease, which might be triggered only by infection with other pathogens. The other way round, MG or MS will aggravate the course of disease caused by these pathogens. The most important synergistic pathogens are *E. coli*, Newcastle disease virus (NDV), avian metapneumovirus and infectious bronchitis virus (IBV). Infections with more than two different respiratory pathogens are common too (Soeripto et al., 1989).

The dynamic is different for MM and MI. Vertically infected turkey breeder hens will start laying infected eggs soon after the onset of lay with increasing rates of up to 60 % at the peak of production, after which rates will decline again. Infection via the respiratory route will rarely and only in young birds lead to vertical transmission (Raviv and Ley, 2013).

Damage caused by the infection with mycoplasmas might be mostly due to the inflammatory host response and less to damage caused directly by the action of the bacteria.

In fact, relative to the importance of mycoplasma infections and the research done on it, few virulence factors have been identified (Ron et al., 2015). Those that have been found include the usual suspects like proteins involved in adhesion and the ability to invade cells (Raviv and Ley, 2013). A very important aspect of infections with mycoplasmas, which is also important for the ability to persistently infect hosts, is immune evasion and immune modulation. Mycoplasmas can evade the immune response by rapidly changing the expression of major antigens and thus their antigenic make-up, a process known as antigenic switching (Noormohammadi, 2007). The importance of those mechanisms for mycoplasmas is illustrated by the fact that in MG at least 10 % of the genome seems to be dedicated to gene families involved in immune evasion (Markham et al., 1993). Mycoplasmas can also modulate the immune system by supressing or stimulating lymphocytes or induction of cytokines.

Some but not all strains of MG, MS and MM are haemagglutinating. The haemagglutinins are important antigens and are also involved in antigenic switching and can be lost during cultivation *in vitro* (Bencina, 2002).

The damage MM does to the skeletal system might be caused by the consumption of biotin by the bacteria and a resulting lack of biotin for the embryo (Bigland and Warenycia, 1978). A similar hypothesis regarding arginine could not be proved.

Clinical signs

The outcome of infection with mycoplasmas depends mainly on route of infection, the infecting strain, age of birds, health status of the bird and, on in the case of respiratory infections, on co-infections with other pathogens. Environmental conditions like temperature, air quality and dust content may also play a role. Colder temperature aggravates the course of the disease and younger birds usually exhibit more severe symptoms.

Generally, turkeys are more susceptible to mycoplasma infections than chickens.

MG: clinical signs are typical for infections of the upper respiratory tract. They include respiratory sounds like coughing and sneezing, nasal and ocular discharge as well as conjunctivitis (Fig. 1). In turkeys, swelling of the infraorbital sinus (Fig. 2) is typical. If birds have airsacculitis, they will exhibit laboured breathing. Feed consumption can decrease and consequently birds will suffer weight loss or a drop in egg production. Morbidity is near 100 % and mortality varies between barely increased to up to 30 %. Signs develop slowly and even after experimental infection with high doses of virulent strains, incubation period can be as long as 3 weeks. Under field conditions, birds can be infected for very long times without showing clinical signs, until stress, particularly at the onset of lay, or infection with other respiratory pathogens trigger the disease. Once they have begun, the symptoms will also take time to resolve and, as indicated by the name CRD, may stay for months if birds are not treated.

MS: infections with MS affect primarily broilers and turkeys between 10 and 20 weeks of age. The incubation period after horizontal infection can be up to 3 weeks. Clinical signs of respiratory infection are minor or inapparent. Clinical signs of tendosynovitis include general depression with ruffled feathers and reluctance to move; joints are swollen followed by lameness. Hocks, footpads, wing joints and the sternal bursa are most frequently involved. Combs of chickens are pale and shrunken. Birds will grow slower and may become emaciated and dehydrated when not able to reach feed and water. In laying hens, egg production may drop by up to 20 % and the eggshell of up to 25 % of the eggs can be thinner, more translucent and have cracks and breaks in the apex (Fig. 3). Birds are slow to recover and synovitis can become chronic. Morbidity is low, usually not exceeding 15 %. Mortality is typically below 1 %.

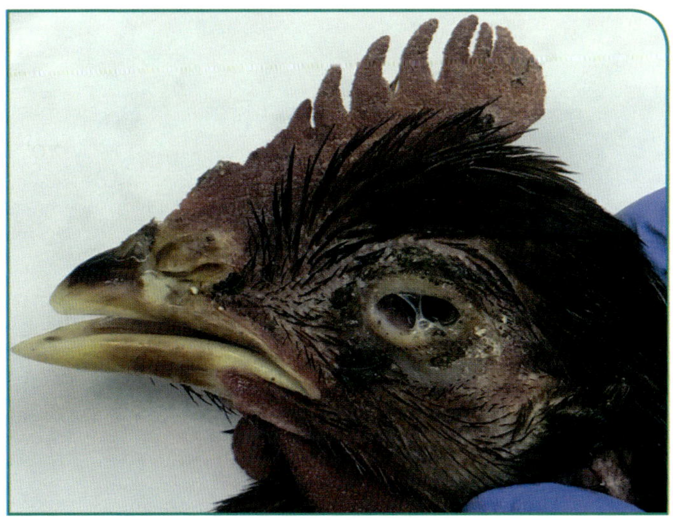

Figure 1. Conjunctivitis after double infection with MG and MS. Image courtesy of Dr. George Cooper and Dr. Manuela Crispo (California Animal Health and Food Safety Laboratory System, Turlock branch).

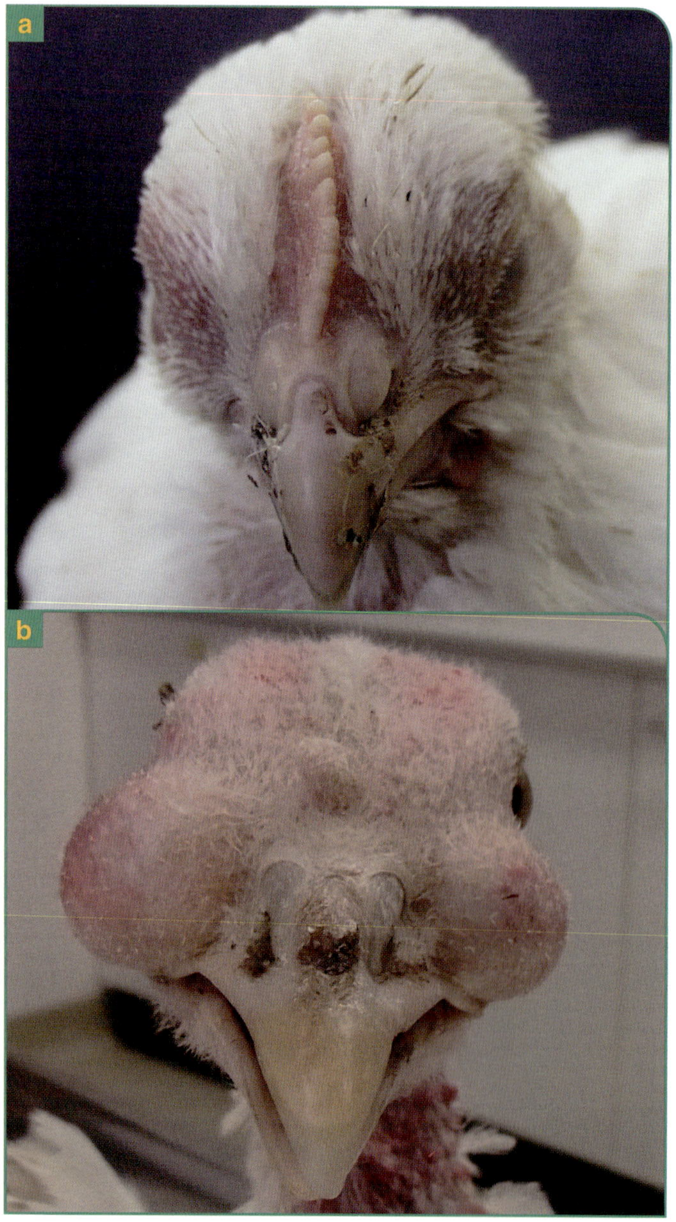

Figure 2. Swelling of the infraorbital sinus of (a) a chicken and (b) a turkey.

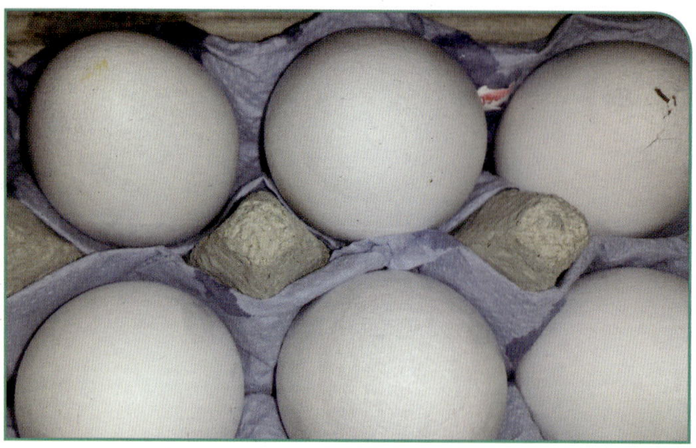

Figure 3. Eggshell apex abnormalities.

MM: horizontal respiratory infection does not cause clinical signs, and poults with airsacculitis due to vertical infections also usually do not show respiratory signs. However, up to 10 % of vertically infected birds can have deformed tarso-metatarsal bones and vertebrae, swollen hocks and abnormal feathering; birds can outgrow the lesions. The condition is also known as TS-65. Late embryo mortality due to infection with MM will decrease hatchability by up to 6 %.

MI: eggs from turkey breeder flocks infected with MI can have a reduced hatchability with embryos typically dying between 18 and 24 days of incubation. Under field conditions, no other clinical signs have been observed, but experimental infection of 1–day-old poults and chicks may result in musculoskeletal lesions and impaired growth.

Post mortem lesions

MG: catarrhal exudate is present throughout the respiratory tract, from the nasal cavity and sinus, through trachea and lungs down to the air sacs. In addition to conjunctivitis, in some cases keratitis recognizable by an opaque cornea may be visible. Facial oedema has also been described. Pneumonia may be present. In more severe cases, the exudate in the air sacs is fibrinous and birds exhibit polyserositis characterized by perihepatitis and pericarditis (Fig 4). If the infection spreads to other organs, it can also cause inflammation there. MG has been associated with salpingitis (Fig. 5) and encephalitis (Wyrzykowski et al., 2013).

Characteristic histopathological lesions are thickening of the mucosal membranes of the affected organs caused by hyperplasia of the mucous glands and infiltration by mononuclear inflammatory cells. Germinal centres are typically hyperplastic. The tracheal epithelium is deciliated. Granulomatous lesions can be present in the lungs.

MS: the respiratory form is characterized by a lack of lesions in the upper respiratory tract, but birds can have severe airsacculitis. In case of tendosynovitis, the exudate is present in the joints (Fig. 6), around the tendons or in the sternal bursa (Fig. 7). In earlier stages of the infection, the exudate appears gray and with a creamy consistence, later it turns caseous. Liver and spleen may be swollen.

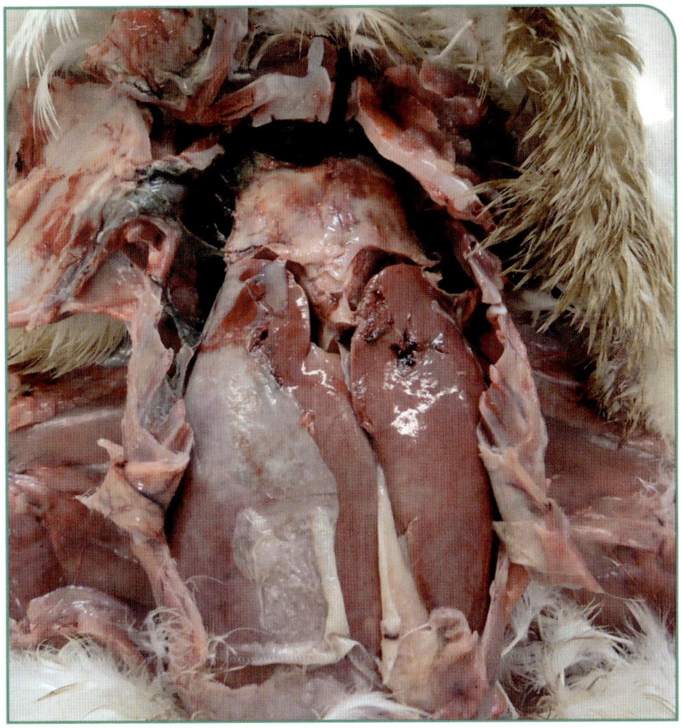

Figure 4. Pericarditis and perihepatitis.

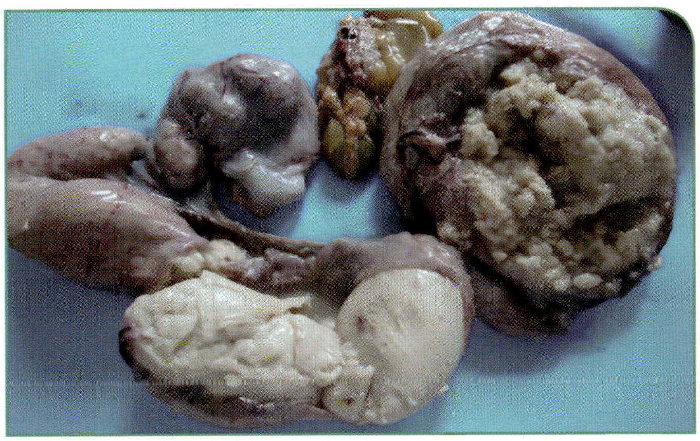

Figure 5. Salpingitis.

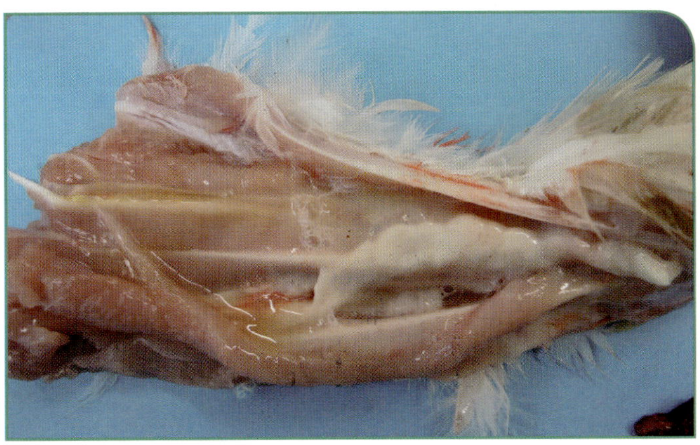

Figure 6. Tendosynovitis.

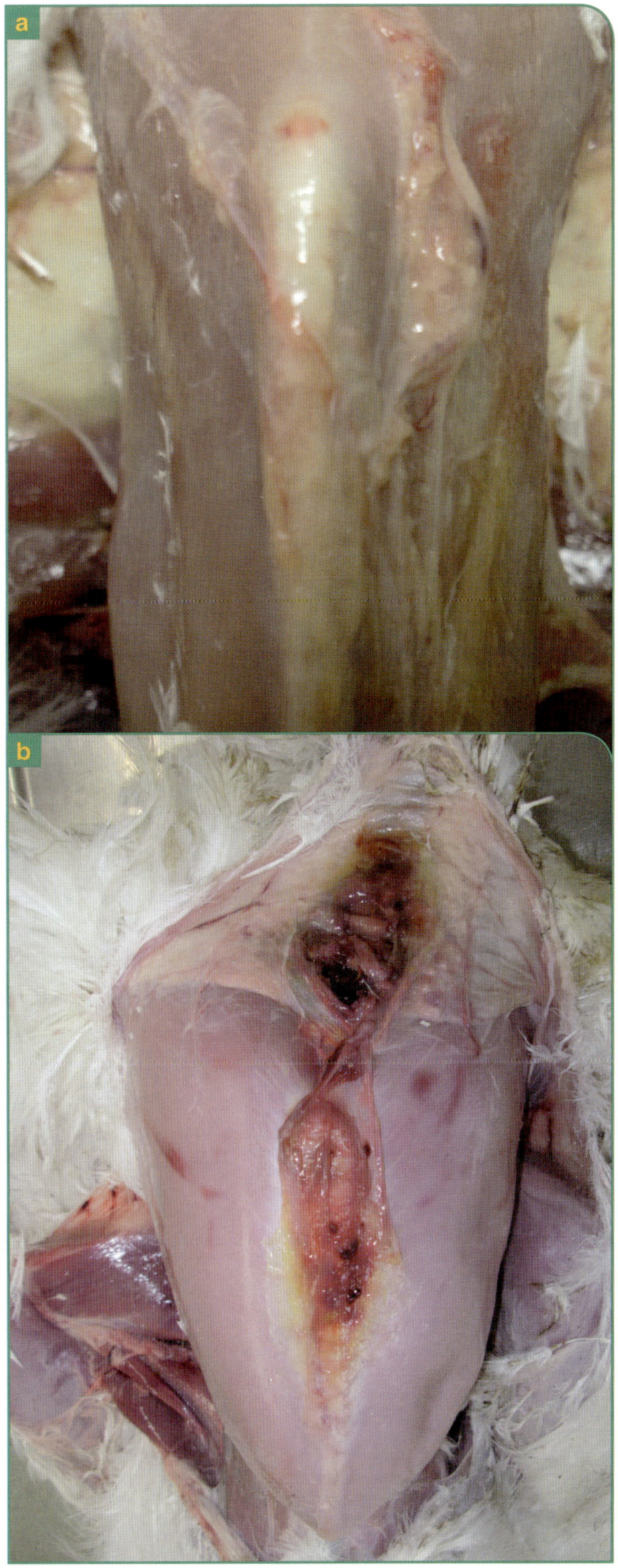

Figure 7. Inflammation of the sternal bursa of (a) a chicken and (b) a turkey.

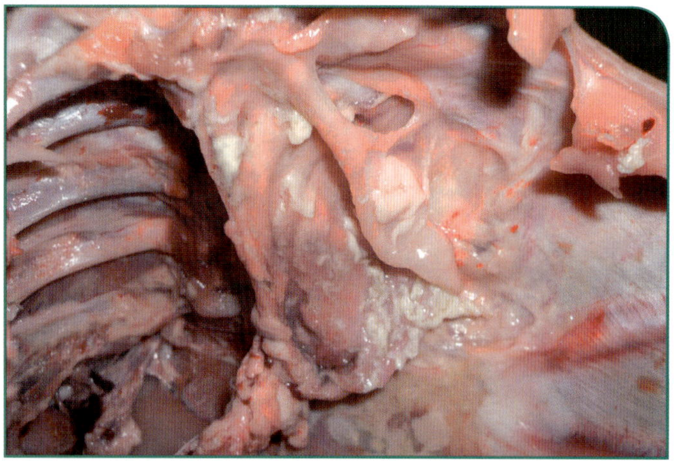

Figure 8. Airsacculitis.

Histopathologically, lesions in the air sac are accumulation of inflammatory cells depending on the stage of the disease, oedema and necrosis. Within the joints and along the tendons, infiltrates of heterophils and fibrin are visible. The synovial membranes are hyperplastic and infiltrated by mononuclear cells.

MM: in flocks with vertically infected poults, up to 25 % of turkeys develop airsacculitis (Fig. 8). The walls are thickened and covered by yellow exudate. Histopathologically, the inflammation is dominated by infiltration with heterophils and accumulation of fibrin. In uncomplicated cases, lesions will disappear by the age of 16 weeks. Lesions in the bones are characterized by a lower cell density in the proliferative zone and abnormal-appearing chondrocytes. Between 6 and 8 weeks of age, lesions in the growth plate regress, but the bone can remain deformed.

MI: as with the clinical signs, no gross lesions have been observed under field conditions, but experimental infection of 1–day-old poults and chicks may result in musculoskeletal lesions like tendosynovitis, chondrodystrophy and deformed bones.

Diagnostic procedures

Suitable samples for isolation or detection of mycoplasmas in the case of disease are exudates of any inflamed organ. Additionally, mycoplasmas can be isolated from the vitelline membrane of hatching eggs or from infected embryos.

For monitoring, oropharyngeal or tracheal swabs are the sample of choice for MG and MS. For MM and MI monitoring, cloacal or vaginal swabs from hens and phallic swabs or semen from toms should be investigated.

During the acute stages of infection, the population of mycoplasma in the respiratory tract is very high. In such cases, 5–10 tracheal or choanal cleft swabs are sufficient for mycoplasma isolation. Due to the low prevalence of infection during persistent infection, it has been recommended to sample between 30 and 100 birds for monitoring in the chronic stage. Even if that is done, the presence of infection within a flock might remain undetected (Raviv and Ley, 2013).

For isolation mycoplasma broth should be inoculated with freshly collected samples. If samples have to be sent to a laboratory, they should be sent using broth as transport medium and be kept at 4 °C for no longer than 24 hours. Shipment on dry ice is also possible if the cold chain is not broken.

Frey's medium (Frey et al., 1968) is most commonly used. The basic version contains casein peptone, soy peptone and yeast extract with 10 % horse or swine serum as well as electrolytes and buffers. Other media that are rich in protein and contain 10–15 % serum can also be suitable. Yeast extract is not absolutely necessary but its addition will usually give better results. For the isolation of MS, the medium has to be substituted with nicotinamide adenine dinucleotide (NAD) and cystein. The addition of phenol red as indicator and glucose will help to determine the right time for passage, if the isolated species metabolizes glucose to acid. MG, MS and MI ferment glucose, while MM does not.

Mycoplasmas grow slowly, so they are easily overgrown by other bacteria or fungi. In order to prevent that, the medium should also contain thallium acetate diluted 1:4000 to inhibit the growth of gram-negative bacteria and 1000 units/ml penicillin to inhibit the growth of gram-positive bacteria. An antimycotic can also be added, e.g. 50 units/ml mycostatin. Because of the considerable toxicity of thallium acetate for humans, its lack of biodegradability and the subsequent accumulation in the environment, it has been suggested to use colistin for the prevention of the growth of gram-negative bacteria instead (Angulo et al., 2003).

The cultures should be incubated at 37 °C aerobically or with increased CO_2 until the phenol red turns yellow, indicating acidity of the medium. If that does not happen after 4 or 5 days, two to three blind passages should be carried out. Then agar plates should be streaked with the broth. Plates have to be incubated in sealed containers or under moist atmosphere to prevent the plates from drying out. Colonies will become visible after 1 to 10 days, depending on the species. Colonies are less than 1 mm in diameter, smooth and round. Their center is dense and elevated, giving them the typical "fried egg appearance" when viewed under a dissecting microscope.

Species identification is usually done by testing the colonies themselves or colony imprints by immunofluorescence, immunoperoxidase reaction or reactions with gene probes.

Other traditional methods are immunodiffusion or growth inhibition by specific antisera. The latter technique can also be used in the case of mixed infections to obtain pure cultures. Differentiation based on biochemical characterization is possible but cumbersome due to the slow growth (Kleven, 2008).

Isolation of mycoplasmas in embryonated chicken eggs after inoculation via the yolk sac route is possible. Inoculation will result in the death of the embryo after 5 to 8 days. Differences in virulence for the embryo exist between strains within one species, but there are not correlated to the virulence of the strain in birds (Glisson and Kleven, 1985; Lockaby et al., 1999).

Today, the standard method for detection of *Mycoplasma* DNA is PCR.

A plethora of assays specific for the various avian mycoplasma species has been published, e.g. by Lierz et al. (2008). Kits are commercially available, and some PCRs are designed to differentiate field strains from vaccine strains (Raviv et al., 2008).

Within MG, MM and especially MI serological different strains exist as shown by haemagglutination inhibition (HI) assay or the use of monoclonal antibodies, but coherent systems for serotyping are missing. Serological differences between MS strains are minor.

Strain differentiation has been done by a variety of methods and there is no a universally applied standard method. The methods include, amongst others, restriction fragment length polymorphism of whole genomes or of individual PCR products, protein banding patterns detected by sodium dodecyl sulfate polyacrylamide gel electrophoresis (SDS-PAGE), random amplification of polymorphic DNA or multilocus sequence typing (MLST).

Detection of antibodies can be used not only for monitoring but also for diagnosis, since in some, but not all, cases antibodies are detectable before the onset of clinical signs. Limitations are that the application of antibiotics can interfere with antibody formation and that respiratory infection of turkeys with MS induces only low antibody titers.

Historically, tube and plate agglutination test and HI have been used as serological tests. The plate agglutination test is prone to non-specific results and sometimes shows cross-reaction between MG and MS. However, the test is quick, inexpensive and highly sensitive, but there are also variations between batches in sensitivity and specificity (Kleven and Levisohn, 1996). False positive reactions are commonly observed in birds vaccinated with inactivated oil-emulsion vaccines against viruses or bacteria. In addition, it is still unknown if infection with non-pathogenic mycoplasmas can cause cross-reactions. Sera showing a positive reaction should be diluted 1:5 and 1:10 with buffer and retested. A titre of 1:5 may be considered suspicious and titres of 1:10 or above regarded as positive.

Sera that produce suspicious results by plate agglutination must be tested by an alternative method such as a HI test. The sensitivity of HI is dependent on how homologue or heterologous the infecting strain and the strain used as antigen are.

Today, the most employed tests are ELISAs, which are sensitive as well as specific. A variety of ELISA kits for detection of antibodies against MG, MS and MM are on the market.

Treatment

In case of clinical respiratory disease, birds should be treated with antibiotics. Treatment will improve clinical signs, lesions and production parameters. It will further decrease the shedding rates, but it will not achieve a total elimination of mycoplasmas.

Suitable antibiotics include tetracyclines, macrolides, tiamulin and fluoroquinolones. Obviously, all antibiotics affecting cell wall synthesis like beta-lactams or colistin will not be effective against mycoplasma. Resistances of mycoplasma against antibiotics can occur, and methods for antimicrobial susceptibility testing have been described. However, they take time due to the slow growth of the bacteria (Hannan, 2000).

Control

Due to the low tenacity of mycoplasmas, routine biosecurity and cleaning and disinfection measures are usually sufficient to prevent horizontal transmission of the bacteria. On the other hand, mycoplasmas easily exploit breaches in biosecurity. Multiple-age flocks and flocks located in areas with high poultry densities are especially at risk.

To prevent vertical introduction into a flock, its parents have to be mycoplasma-free; thus, the production pyramid needs to be cleaned from the top.

To do that, extensive eradication programmes including serological testing of birds high up in the pyramid have been done to prevent mycoplasma introduction through primary and commercial breeder flocks. To break the vertical transmission cycle and obtain a sufficient number of mycoplasma-negative birds to start building mycoplasma-free flocks, these programmes were complemented by treatment of hatching eggs. Antibiotics were applied by egg injection or by dipping the eggs into antibiotic solutions, taking advantage of differences in temperature or pressure to deliver the antibiotic inside the egg. Alternatively, eggs were heated to a temperature-time combination, for example 46.1 °C over 12–14 hours that killed mycoplasma. On the downside, none of these methods is 100 % effective and some reduce hatchability for more than 10 % or carry the risk of another bacterial contamination. While these programmes have succeeded, close monitoring by PCR or ELISA of breeder flocks is necessary, because an unnoticed infection in those flocks would affect a vast number of progeny flocks. Suggested monitoring intervals are every 2 weeks for chickens and every 3 weeks for turkeys (Raviv and Ley, 2013).

A variety of vaccines against mycoplasmas is commercially available.

Similar to treatment with antibiotics, vaccination will prevent or lessen clinical signs and lesions, improve production parameters and decrease the shedding rate in the case of infection. Vaccination will not prevent infection or shedding, including vertical transmission. Additionally, it will interfere with serological monitoring.

For MG, killed and live vaccines are available. The benefits of killed MG vaccines have been questioned, especially regarding the need for individual application and for a booster vaccine (Raviv and Ley, 2013). However, vaccination with bacterins provides good protection against egg production losses. Under field conditions, an increase of up to 19 eggs per hen more has been observed in vaccinated flocks. Other potential benefits include improved feed conversion and reductions of medication costs.

Live MG vaccines for chickens contain one of three strains, namely F-strain, 6/85 or temperature-sensitive ts-11. These strains differ regarding their residual virulence, the quality of the protection they offer and, importantly, their potential of transmission, including vertical transmission. Their advantages and disadvantages have been discussed in detail by Raviv and Ley (2013). Their use in turkeys is not recommended: in the case of F-strain because it is too virulent in this species, while the other two strains do not induce significant protection. A recombinant fowlpox vaccine expressing MG antigen is also available (Zhang et al., 2010). Other vaccine strains have been tested, but seem not to be commercially available (Papazisi et al., 2002; Ferguson et al., 2004).

For MS, strain MS-1 and temperature-sensitive strain MS-H as well as a killed vaccine are commercially available in some markets. These vaccines are only for chickens.

There are no vaccines against MM and MI.

References

ANGULO AF, JACOBS MV, VAN DAMME EHA, AKKERMANS AM, DE KRUIJFF-KROESEN I AND BRUGMAN J. Colistin sulfate as a suitable substitute of thallium acetate in culture media intended for mycoplasma detection and culture. *Biologicals*. 2003; 31, 161–163.

BENCINA D. Haemagglutinins of pathogenic avian mycoplasmas. *Avian Pathology*. 2002; 31, 535–547.

BIGLAND CH AND WARENYCIA MW. Effects of biotin, folic acid, and pantothenic acid on the growth of *Mycoplasma meleagridis*, a turkey pathogen. *Poultry Science*. 1978; 57, 611–618.

CHRISTENSEN NH, YAVARI CA, MCBAIN AJ AND BRADBURY JM. Investigations into the survival of *Mycoplasma gallisepticum*, *Mycoplasma synoviae* and *Mycoplasma iowae* on materials found in the poultry house environment. *Avian Pathology*. 1994; 23, 127–143.

FERGUSON NM, LEITING VA AND KLEVEN SH. Safety and efficacy of the avirulent *Mycoplasma gallisepticum* strain K5054 as a live vaccine in poultry. *Avian Diseases*. 2004; 48, 91–99.

FREY ML, HANSON RP AND ANDRSON DP. A medium for the isolation of avian mycoplasmas. *American Journal of Veterinary Research*. 1968; 29, 2163–2171.

GLISSON JR AND KLEVEN SH. *Mycoplasma gallisepticum* vaccination: further studies on egg transmission and egg production. *Avian Diseases*. 1985; 29, 408–415.

HANNAN PCT. Guidelines and recommendations for antimicrobial minimum inhibitory concentration (MIC) testing against veterinary mycoplasma species. *Veterinary Research*. 2000; 31, 373–395.

KLEVEN SH. Mycoplasmosis. In: A laboratory manual for the isolation, identification and characterization of avian pathogens, L Duforu-Zavala, DE Swayne, JR Glisson, JE Pearson, WM Reed, MW Jackwood and PR Woolcock, eds. Jacksonville, FA: The American Association of Avian Pathologists. 2008; pp. 59–64.

KLEVEN SH, FLETCHER OJ AND DAVIS RB. Influence of strain of *Mycoplasma synoviae* and route of infection on development of synovitis or airsacculitis in broilers. *Avian Diseases*. 1975; 19, 126–135.

KLEVEN SH AND LEVISOHN S. Mycoplasma infections of poultry. In: Molecular and diagnostic procedures in mycoplasmology, vol II. (J.G. Tully & S. Razin-Eds). Academic Press, New York. 1996; pp. 283–292.

LIERZ M, HAGEN N, LUESCHOW D AND HAFEZ HM. Use of polymerase chain reactions to detect *Mycoplasma gallisepticum*, *Mycoplasma imitans*, *Mycoplasma iowae*, *Mycoplasma meleagridis* and *Mycoplasma synoviae* in birds of prey. *Avian Pathology: journal of the WVPA*. 2008; 37, 471–476.

LOCKABY SB, HOERR FJ, KLEVEN SH AND LAUERMAN LH. Pathogenicity of *Mycoplasma synoviae* in chicken embryos. *Avian Diseases*. 1999; 43, 331–337.

Markham PF, Glew MD, Whithear KG and Walker ID. Molecular cloning of a member of the gene family that encodes pMGA, a hemagglutinin of *Mycoplasma gallisepticum*. *Infection and Immunity*. 1993; 61, 903–909.

Noormohammadi AH. Role of phenotypic diversity in pathogenesis of avian mycoplasmosis. *Avian Pathology*. 2007; 36, 439–444.

Papazisi L, Silbart LK, Frasca Jr. S, Rood D, Liao X, Gladd M, Javed MA and Geary SJ. A modified live *Mycoplasma gallisepticum* vaccine to protect chickens from respiratory disease. *Vaccine*. 2002; 20, 3709–3719.

Raviv Z and Ley DH. *Mycoplasma gallisepticum* infection. In: Diseases of poultry, DE Swayne, JR Glisson, LR McDougald, LK Nolan, DL Suarez and V Nair, eds. Ames, Iowa: Iowa State Press. 2013; pp. 877–893.

Raviv Z, Callison SA, Ferguson-Noel N and Kleven SH. Strain differentiating real-time PCR for *Mycoplasma gallisepticum* live vaccine evaluation studies. *Veterinary Microbiology*. 2008; 129, 179–187.

Roberts DH and McDaniel JW. Mechanism of egg transmission of *Mycoplasma gallisepticum*. *Journal of Comparative Pathology*. 1967; 77, 439–442.

Ron M, Gorelick-Ashkenazi A, Levisohn S, Nir-Paz R, Geary SJ, Tulman E, Lysnyansky I and Yogev D. *Mycoplasma gallisepticum* in vivo induced antigens expressed during infection in chickens. *Veterinary Microbiology*. 2015; 175, 265–274.

Sasipreeyajan J, Halvorson DA and Newman JA. Effect of *Mycoplasma gallisepticum* bacterin on egg-*transmission* and egg production. *Avian Diseases*. 1987; 31, 776–781.

Soeripto, Whithear K, Cottew G and Harrigan K. Virulence and transmissibility of *Mycoplasma gallisepticum*. *Australian Veterinary Journal*. 1989; 66, 65–72.

Wyrzykowski B, Albaric O, Moreau S, Nguyen F, Fleurance R, Belluco S, Wyers M and Colle M-A. Retrospective study of *Mycoplasma gallisepticum* meningoencephalitis in six turkey flocks in western France. *Journal of Comparative Pathology*. 2013; 148, 173–177.

Zhang GZ, Zhang R, Zhao HL, Wang XT, Zhang SP, Li XJ, Qin CZ, Lv CM, Zhao JX and Zhou JF. A safety assessment of a fowlpox-vectored *Mycoplasma gallisepticum* vaccine in chickens. *Poultry Science*. 2010; 89, 1301–1306.

9 Chlamydiosis

Avian chlamydiosis is a usually systemic disease of birds that is caused by *Chlamydia psittaci*. In poultry, turkeys and ducks are most susceptible, but recent studies show that there is also a high prevalence of infection in chickens. *C. psittaci* can also infect humans causing human chlamydiosis. The disease of humans and birds was referred to as psittacosis, when it occurred in parrots or if it had been contracted from parrots, or as ornithosis, when occurring in fowl or if it had been contracted from fowl. Today, this distinction is considered to be obsolete, because the severity depends on the particular interaction of host and infecting strain and not on the host species alone. There is also no correlation between the host from which humans acquired the infection and the severity of disease.

Humans can get infected by inhalation of aerosols when handling infected birds. Thus, veterinarians are at risk when visiting poultry houses with infected birds or when doing post-mortem examination on them. Other professions at risk are poultry farmers, workers in processing plants and laboratory staff. Human chlamydiosis is an influenza-like systemic disease, often with pneumonia, but depending on the infecting strain the infection can also be subclinical. The prognosis is good if treated timely and adequately. Transmission between humans is rare.

Aetiology

Classification of *C. psittaci* has changed twice in the last 20 years. Between 1999 and 2009, the family Chlamydiaceae was divided into two genera, *Chlamydia* and *Chlamydophila*, based on the sequences of the ribosomal RNA genes (Everett et al., 1999). *C. psittaci* was grouped into the latter genus and thus named *Chlamydophila psittaci*. Taking into account more genes than just the ribosomal RNA genes, the change was reversed in 2009 and *Chlamydia* is again the only recognized species in the family (Stephens et al., 2009).

Nine types of *C. psittaci* are recognized. They were originally defined as serotypes, but nowadays are determined by molecular biological methods (Geens et al., 2005). Types A to F and E/B have been isolated from various bird species; the other two serotypes M56 and WC have only been found in mammals (Vanrompay, 2013). Other *Chlamydia* spp. including *C. pecorum*, *C. trachomatis*, *C. abortus* and others have also been isolated from birds. Additionally, new species occurring in birds have been recently described (Vorimore et al., 2013; Sachse et al., 2014).

Chlamydia have a gram-negative cell wall. They are obligatory intracellular and take one of three different morphological forms during different stages of their life cycle (AbdelRahman and Belland, 2005). Outside the host cell, they are small round cells, about 0.2–0.3 µm in diameter and are called elementary bodies (EBs). EBs are electron dense and metabolically inactive, but infectious. Inside of cells, chlamydia are present as reticular bodies (RBs), which are about 0.5–2.0 µm in diameter. RBs are metabolically active, but lack some pathways like the pentose and citric cycles, which makes them dependent on the host cell. RBs divide by binary fission.

Chlamydia are susceptible to commonly used disinfectants. In the environment, they remain infective for several days.

Pathogenesis and transmission

Chlamydia infect their hosts mainly via the respiratory route by inhalation of aerosols or dust; infection by the faecal-oral route is also possible. Mites and flies might serve as vectors, but probably are of little importance. As indicated above, the host spectrum is very wide; the latest count identified 465 bird species from 30 orders (Kaleta and Taday, 2003), and it has been stated that virtually every bird species might become infected.

Chapter co-authored by [illegible] L. Shivaprasad (California Animal Health and Food Safety Laboratory System, Tulare branch).

There is some correlation between type, host and severity of disease, even though there is no strict host specificity of the types.

Most cases in turkeys are caused by infection with types B and D, and cases due to infection with type B are typically less severe than cases due to infection with type D. Severe disease after infection with type C and milder disease after infection with types A or E have also been described. Based on epidemiology, it is assumed that chlamydiosis is not endemic in turkeys, but every outbreak is due to a new introduction. Regarding the natural reservoirs, serovars B and E are thought to be endemic in pigeons and doves, which can be persistently infected with these types without developing disease. An equivalent host that might serve as reservoir of type D is not known, but it has been postulated that there is one. Types C and E/B are associated with water fowl; types A and F with psittacines. Mammals do not play a role as reservoirs, because strains that naturally occur in mammals are distinct and do not cause disease in birds.

Vertical transmission has been demonstrated, but there is no indication that it plays a major role in the epidemiology of avian chlamydiosis.

EBs attach to epithelial cells and are taken up by endocytosis in membrane vacuoles. Chlamydia prevent fusion of the vacuoles with lysosomes. The vacuoles are visible as inclusion bodies. Inside the vacuoles, EBs develop into RBs by initiation of transcription and translation of genes, changes in the cell wall and general growth. RBs undergo several rounds of cell division after which they will transform into EBs. Strains with higher virulence can also escape from their vacuole and multiply in the cytoplasm. After about 2 days, when several hundred EBs have been formed, the host cell lyses, releasing the EBs. Alternative outcomes are exocytosis of the EBs and survival of the cell or persistent infection of the host cell. Persistent infection can be reactivated leading to shedding of chlamydia and clinical disease when the host is stressed (AbdelRahman and Belland, 2005).

After replication in the epithelial cells in the upper respiratory tract, infection moves down to the lower respiratory tract. From there, chlamydia spread within monocytes in the blood as well as free in the plasma to other organs, most importantly the digestive tract, but also liver, spleen, kidney or other organs. In these organs, chlamydia infect epithelial cells and macrophages (Vanrompay et al., 1995a).

The mechanisms by which *C. psittaci* manipulates the cell in order to prevent the fusion of its vacuole with lysosomes, to navigate the vacuole close to cell organelles and to acquire ATP and other metabolites are partially known, as is its interaction with the immune system (Knittler et al., 2014). There is no information on virulence factors responsible for the variation in course of disease in the different host species.

Clinical signs

As discussed above, the course of disease is mostly determined by the combination of host species and infecting chlamydia strain. Incubation period also depends on the virulence of the strain; it can be as short as 5–10 days for virulent strains, but up to 8 weeks after infection with strains with lower virulence. Additionally, younger birds tend to be more susceptible than older ones.

Clinical signs in turkeys indicate a systemic disease involving the respiratory and digestive tract. They include general depression and reduced feed consumption, which will lead to chachexia in severe chronic cases. Respiratory signs are characterized by conjunctivitis, nasal and ocular discharge and laboured breathing. The nasal gland can be swollen and form a noticeable swelling (bump) over one or both eyes, which might be the only clinical sign (Fig. 1). Yellow-green, gelatinous diarrhoea shows involvement of the digestive tract.

Morbidity after infection with virulent strains can go up to 80 %, while after infection with less virulent strains only up to 20 %. Mortality can be up to 30 % and 5 %, respectively. Egg production in turkey hens can drop up to 20 %.

Clinical signs in ducks are similar. Additionally, young ducks often develop central nervous signs like uncoordinated movements and trembling. Co-infection with *Salmonella* can significantly aggravate the disease.

Infected chickens usually do not show clinical signs. If they do, the signs remain mostly restricted to the respiratory tract.

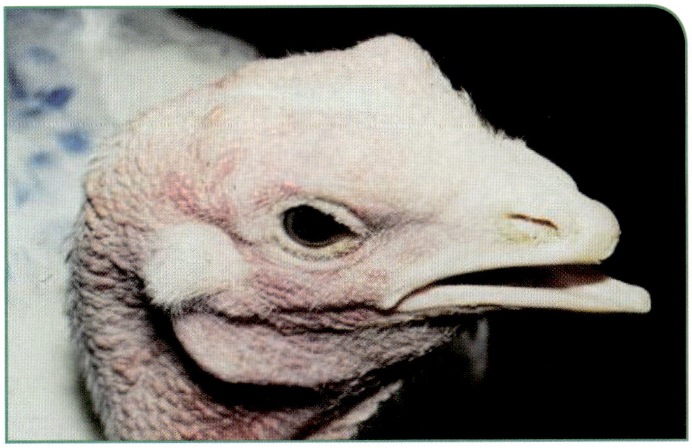

Figure 1. Swelling above the left eye due to inflammation of the nasal gland infected with chlamydia. Image courtesy of Dr. H.L. Shivaprasad (California Animal Health and Food Safety Laboratory System, Tulare branch).

Post mortem lesions

Typical gross lesions include polyserositis, pneumonia and enlarged spleen and liver. Polyserositis is characterized by fibrinous exudate filling the air sacs and covering heart, liver and spleen. The air sac wall and pericardium are thickened. The lungs are dark red and congested. The swollen spleen is softer than usual and can be mottled, and the enlarged liver is friable and greenish discoloured. In the acute stage, birds also have catarrhal enteritis. Nasal glands can be enlarged with brownish discolouration (Fig. 2).

Histopathologically, the exudate covering the inflamed serosae contains large amounts of fibrin and macrophages and only few lymphocytes and heterophils. Pneumonia is characterized by similar exudate in the tertiary bronchi and respiratory tubules; additionally, there might be areas of necrosis. Most prominent lesions in the spleen are reticuloendothelial cell hyperplasia and necrotic areas. In the liver, sinusoids are dilated and infiltrated with inflammatory cells; the Kupffer cells are swollen, and necrotic hepatocytes and foci of necrosis are present throughout the organ. Additionally, there might be myocarditis. In the nasal glands, there is a disruption of the normal architecture due to severe infiltration of heterophils in acute stages and mononuclear cells infiltration in later stages (Fig. 3). In all organs, blood vessels are congested.

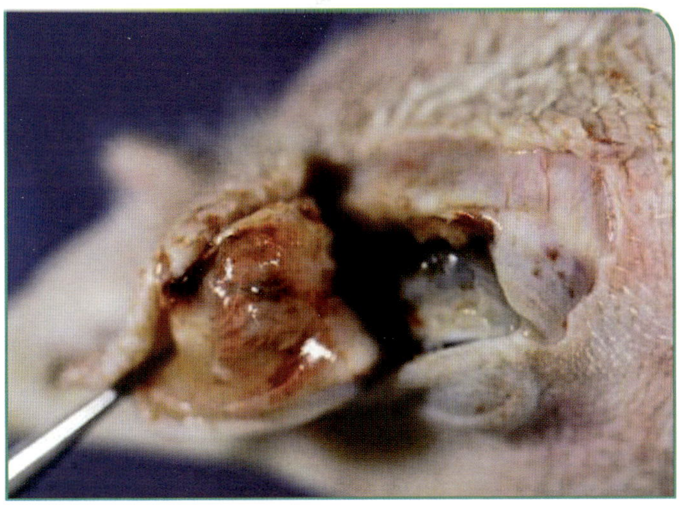

Figure 2. Swelling and brownish discolouration of the nasal gland due to infection with chlamydia. Image courtesy of Dr. H.L. Shivaprasad (California Animal Health and Food Safety Laboratory System, Tulare branch).

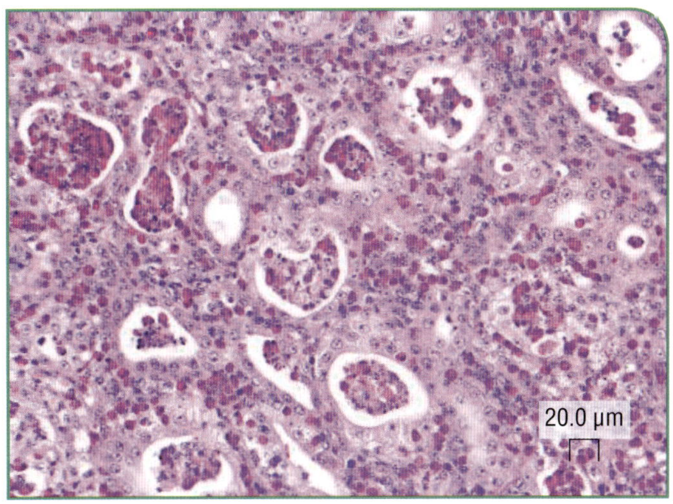

Figure 3. Nasal gland with severe infiltration of heterophils and distortion of the glands due to infection with chlamydia. Image courtesy of Dr. H.L. Shivaprasad (California Animal Health and Food Safety Laboratory System, Tulare branch).

Diagnostic procedures

When avian chlamydiosis is suspected, rigorous safety precautions in accordance with local regulations have to be taken to avoid infection of pathologists and laboratory staff.

A quick method to substantiate a presumptive diagnosis is staining impression smears of livers, spleens or the exudate. Recommended stains include Giemsa stain, which will stain EBs blue, as well as Gimenez or Stamp stains, which will stain EBs red (Fig. 4). Even though chlamydia have a gram-negative cell wall, Gram stain is of no practical value. Immunohistochemistry is another method that can be used to diagnose chlamidya readily (Fig. 5).

From dead birds, all organs with lesions can be sampled for isolation or detection by PCR. In live birds, conjunctival, choanal and cloacal swabs are suitable.

For PCR, all three sites can be sampled using the same swab; for isolation, a cleaner sample without bacterial contamination from the cloaca is preferable. Growth of contaminating bacteria can also be prevented by adding aminoglycoside antibiotics or vancomycin and fungicides to the transport medium. Sucrose-phosphate-glutamic acid (SPG) buffer with 10 % serum is a suitable transport medium (Spencer and Johnson, 1983).

C. psittaci can be isolated in a variety of mammalian and avian cell lines, including frequently used HeLa and Buffalo Green Monkey cells. Sensitivity can be increased by suppressing eukaryotic cell division with suitable chemicals and by centrifugating the inoculum onto the cell monolayer. Chlamydia can be detected in the cell cultures by immunofluorescence, aforementioned stains or PCR. Alternatively, embryonated specific pathogen-free (SPF) eggs from chickens not receiving antibiotics that are active against chlamydia can be inoculated into the yolk sac. Infected embryos will die after 3 to 10 days. One or two blind passages might be necessary. Impression smears of the yolk sac can be used for detection of chlamydia (Vanrompay, 2013).

Species identification and typing can be done either by serology using specific antisera or monoclonal antibodies, or by PCR and sequencing the intergenic spacer separating the 16S and 23S rRNA genes or the outer membrane protein A (Everett et al., 1999; Geens et al., 2005).

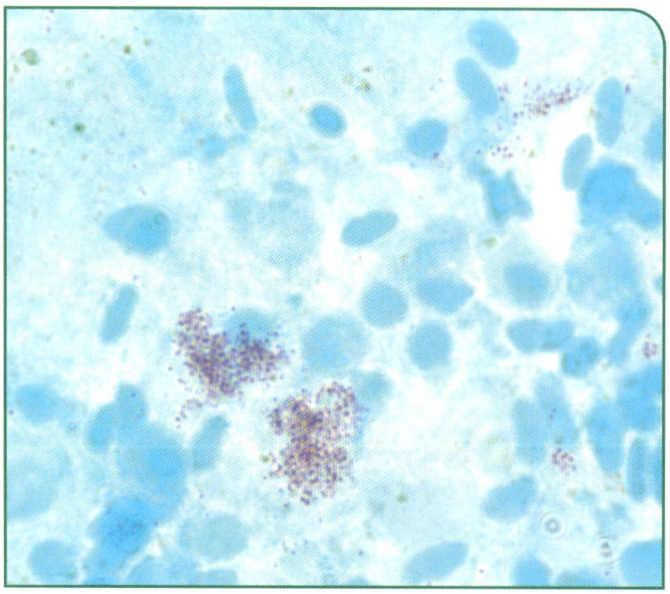

Figure 4. Organ smear stained with Stamp stain. Note two cells with formed but not yet released EB and extracellular EB nearby. Image courtesy of Dr. Sarah Brüggemann-Schwarze (Institute for Poultry Diseases, Freie Universität Berlin).

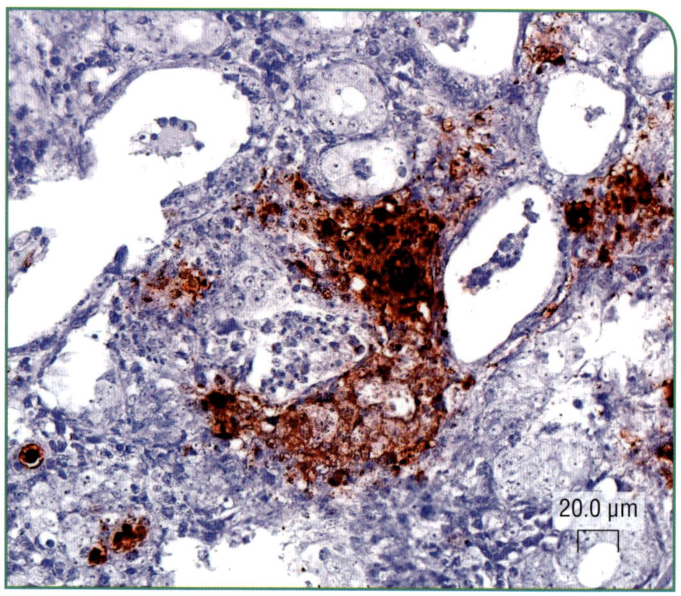

Figure 5. Immunohistochemistry showing brown chlamydia antigen in the cytoplasm of a few glands and inflammatory cells. Image courtesy of Dr. H.L. Shivaprasad (California Animal Health and Food Safety Laboratory System, Tulare branch).

PCR assays for direct detection in clinical samples have also been published, but seem to have a lower sensitivity than isolation in cell culture. Kits to detect chlamydia antigen directly in clinical samples are on the market, but lack in sensitivity and specificity (Sting et al., 2006). Recently, a microarray-based method for genotyping of chlamydia directly from tissue samples has been described (Sachse and Ruettger, 2015). In addition to sampling birds, air sampling has been used to monitor flocks and processing plants in order to minimize risk for workers (Dickx et al., 2010).

Detection of antibodies can be used for diagnosis if the antibody titer increases fourfold or more within a period of 2 weeks.

Frequently used tests are complement fixation, which is regarded as the gold standard, latex agglutination and elementary body agglutination, ELISA as well as indirect immunofluorescence (Vanrompay, 2013).

Treatment

Chlamydia are usually susceptible to sulphonamides, tetracyclines, fluoroquinolones and erythromycin. Interestingly, even though they are gram-negative, they are also partially susceptible to penicillin and other beta-lactams; the reasons behind that are not fully understood (Ghuysen and Goffin, 1999).

The recommended treatment is chlortetracycline or doxycycline, which has some practical advantages over chlortetracycline.

The drugs should be given in the feed for at least 2 weeks, but even after prolonged treatment, it is questionable if a flock will clear the infection. To make the treatment more effective, reinfection should be minimized by concurrent disinfection, if possible, and the immune system should be strengthened by avoiding to stress the birds, supplementing vitamins and electrolytes as well as by increasing the ambient temperature (Vanrompay et al., 1995b). In uncomplicated cases, the disease might resolve without therapy (Shivaprasad et al., 2015). An important aspect of treatment is to stop shedding of chlamydia so that farm workers and, if the birds are allowed to be slaughtered, workers at the processing plant are not put at risk.

Legal regulations have to be observed. These might include reporting the disease to the appropriate authorities, following specific treatments and monitoring for their success as well as imposing a quarantine restricting movement of live birds and carcasses.

Control

Control of avian chlamydiosis has to rely on preventing the introduction of the causative agents into flocks. Among the common biosecurity measures, preventing contact with wild birds, especially pigeons that are reservoirs of chlamydia, is most important. Flocks with outdoor-access are at special risk (Shivaprasad et al., 2015).

Commercial vaccines against chlamydia are not available and attempts to develop a vaccine were remarkably unsuccessful.

Recently, a herpesvirus of turkeys (HVT) vectored recombinant vaccine was shown to provide partial protection for experimentally infected chickens (Liu et al., 2015).

References

AbdelRahman YM and Belland RJ. The chlamydial developmental cycle. *FEMS Microbiology Reviews*. 2005; 29, 949–959.

Dickx V, Geens T, Deschuyffeleer T, Tyberghien L, Harkinezhad T, Beeckman DSA, Braeckman L and Vanrompay D. *Chlamydophila psittaci* zoonotic risk assessment in a chicken and turkey slaughterhouse. *Journal of Clinical Microbiology*. 2010; 48, 3244–3250.

Everett KDE, Bush RM and Andersen AA. Emended description of the order Chlamydiales, proposal of Parachlamydiaceae fam. nov. and Simkaniaceae fam. nov., each containing one monotypic genus, revised taxonomy of the family Chlamydiaceae, including a new genus and five new species, and standards for the identification of organisms. *International Journal of Systematic and Evolutionary Microbiology*. 1999; 49, 415–440.

Geens T, Desplanques A, Van Loock M, Bönner BM, Kaleta EF, Magnino S, Andersen AA, Everett KDE and Vanrompay D. Sequencing of the *Chlamydophila psittaci* ompA gene reveals a new genotype, E/B, and the need for a rapid discriminatory genotyping method. *Journal of Clinical Microbiology*. 2005; 43, 2456–2461.

Ghuysen J-M and Goffin C. Lack of cell wall peptidoglycan versus penicillin sensitivity: new insights into the chlamydial anomaly. *Antimicrobial Agents and Chemotherapy*. 43, 2339–2344.

Kaleta EF and Taday EMA. Avian host range of *Chlamydophila* spp. based on isolation, antigen detection and serology. *Avian Pathology*. 2003; 32, 435–462.

Knittler MR, Berndt A, Böcker S, Dutow P, Hänel F, Heuer D, Kägebein D, Klos A, Koch S, Liebler-Tenorio E, Osterman C, Reinhold P, Saluz HP, Schöfl G, Sehnert P and Sachse K. *Chlamydia psittaci*: New insights into genomic diversity, clinical pathology, host–pathogen interaction and anti-bacterial immunity. *International Journal of Medical Microbiology*. 2014; 304, 877–893.

Liu S, Sun W, Chu J, Huang X, Wu Z, Yan M, Zhang Q, Zhao P, Igietseme JU, Black CM, He C and Li Y. Construction of recombinant HVT expressing PmpD, and immunological evaluation against *Chlamydia psittaci* and Marek's Disease Virus. *PLoS ONE*. 2015; 10: e0124992.

Sachse K and Ruettger A. Rapid microarray-based genotyping of *Chlamydia* spp. strains from clinical tissue samples. In: Veterinary Infection Biology: Molecular Diagnostics and High-Throughput Strategies, MV Cunha and J Inácio, eds. Springer New York. 2015; pp. 391–400.

Sachse K, Laroucau K, Riege K, Wehner S, Dilcher M, Creasy HH, Weidmann M, Myers G, Vorimore F, Vicari N, Magnino S, Liebler-Tenorio E, Ruettger A, Bavoli PM, Hufert FT, Roselló-Móra R and Marz M. Evidence for the existence of two new members of the family Chlamydiaceae and proposal of *Chlamydia avium* sp. nov. and *Chlamydia gallinacea* sp. nov. *Systematic and Applied Microbiology*. 2014; 37, 79–88.

Shivaprasad HL, Carnaccini S, Bland M, Aaziz R, Moeller R and Laroucau K. An unusual outbreak of chlamydiosis in commercial turkeys involving the nasal glands. *Avian Diseases*. 2015; 59, 315–322.

Spencer WN and Johnson FW. Simple transport medium for the isolation of *Chlamydia psittaci* from clinical material. *Veterinary Record*. 1983; 113, 535–536.

Stephens RS, Myers G, Eppinger M and Bavoil PM. Divergence without difference: phylogenetics and taxonomy of Chlamydia resolved. *FEMS Immunology and Medical Microbiology*. 2009; 55, 115–119.

Sting R, Lerke E, Hotzel H, Jodas S, Popp C and Hafez HM. Comparative studies on detection of *Chlamydophila psittaci* and *Chlamydophila abortus* in meat turkey flocks using cell culture, ELISA, and PCR. *DTW. Deutsche. Tierärztliche Wochenschrift*. 2006; 113, 50–54.

Vanrompay D. Avian chlamydiosis. In: Diseases of Poultry, DE Swayne, JR Glisson, LR McDougald, LK Nolan, DL Suarez and V Nair, eds. Ames, Iowa: Iowa State Press. 2013; pp. 1055–1073.

Vanrompay D, Mast J, Ducatelle R, Haesebrouck F and Goddeeris B. *Chlamydia psittaci* in turkeys: pathogenesis of infections in avian serovars A, B and D. *Veterinary Microbiology*. 1995a; 47, 245–256.

Vanrompay D, Ducatelle R and Haesebrouck F. *Chlamydia psittaci* infections: a review with emphasis on avian chlamydiosis. *Veterinary Microbiology*. 1995b; 45, 93–119.

Vorimore F, Hsia R, Huot-Creasy H, Bastian S, Deruyter L, Passet A, Sachse K, Bavoil P, Myers G and Laroucau K. Isolation of a new chlamydia species from the feral sacred ibis (Threskiornis aethiopicus): *Chlamydia ibidis*. *PLoS ONE*. 2013; 8, e74823.

10 Necrotic enteritis

Necrotic enteritis (NE) is a multifactorial disease, but its most important factor is colonization with large numbers of *Clostridium perfringens*. There are also instances in which other *Clostridia* spp. like *C. colinum*, *C. sordellii* and *C. difficile* have been associated with NE-like disease (Uzal et al., 2016). NE is mainly a disease of broilers and to a lesser extent of meat turkeys, but it has also been described in other bird species.

The condition occurs worldwide and its importance is rising everywhere, where the use of antimicrobial growth promoters has been banned or has been voluntarily ceased.

C. perfringens can cause several clinical or subclinical manifestations and lesions in poultry, including necrotic enteritis, necrotic dermatitis, cholangiohepatitis as well as gizzard erosions. Additionally, *C. perfringens* can be responsible for food poisoning in humans (Songer, 2010).

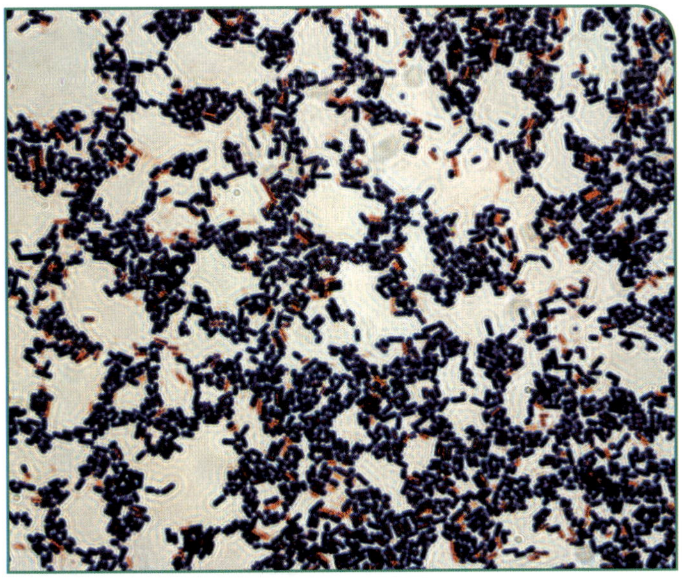

Figure 1. *Clostridium perfringens* cells. Gram stain. Image courtesy of Dr. Sarah Brüggemann-Schwarze (Institute for Poultry Diseases, Freie Universität Berlin).

Aetiology

C. perfringens is a gram-positive, rod-shaped bacterium. Its cells measure 0.6–2.4 x 1.3–19.0 µm (Fig. 1). *C. perfringens* is a strict anaerobe and can form spores, but does so rarely *in vitro*. If spores are present, they are oval, centrally or subterminally located and large and extending the cell. The majority of strains has a capsule. *C. perfringens* is notable for having an extremely short generation time of 6.3 minutes under optimal conditions (Labbe and Huang, 1995).

The genus *Clostridium* is the most important genus within the class Clostridia. It contains several notable pathogens causing disease in various hosts, like. *C. botulinum*, which is covered in the following chapter.

Based on the ability to produce one or several toxins, which are summarily referred to as major toxins, five types designated A–E are differentiated based on the synthesis of four major lethal toxins: alpha, beta, epsilon, and iota (Table 1). Isolates causing NE in poultry usually belong to type A. Sometimes Type C is found, very rarely other types (Opengart and Songer, 2013). Strains causing NE are more closely related to each other than non-virulent isolates (Lacey et al., 2016).

Table 1. Production of major toxins by *C. perfringens* types A–E.

TYPE	TOXINS PRODUCED
A	Alpha
B	Alpha, beta and epsilon
C	Alpha and beta
D	Alpha and epsilon
E	Alpha and iota

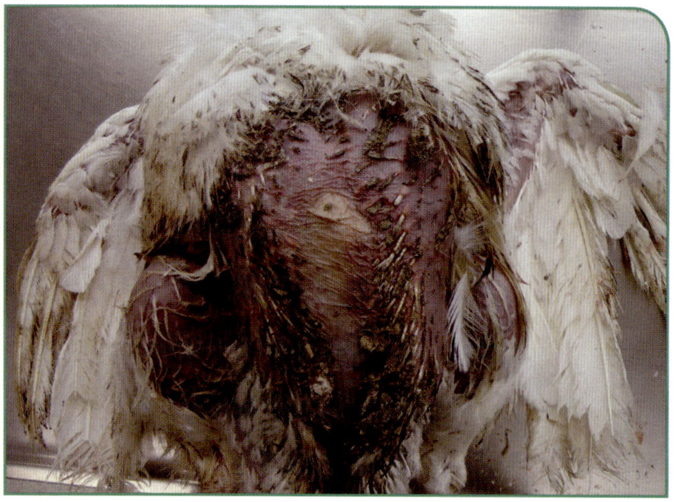

Figure 2. Gangrenous dermatitis associated with *Clostridium perfringens*.

Similar diseases in various hosts are also associated with one or more of the types. In addition to those specific diseases, *C. perfringens* frequently causes wound infections in all hosts. In poultry it is one major causative agent in gangrenous dermatitis (Fig. 2).

Pathogenesis and transmission

C. perfringens is ubiquitous. It has been isolated from the intestines "of virtually every animal that has been investigated" (Rainey et al., 2015) and can be considered to be part of the normal intestinal flora of the lower intestine. The small intestine should harbour only low number of *C. perfringens* and disease is usually associated with 10^6 to 10^8 cfu/g ingesta (Timbermont et al., 2011). Bacteria are shed in the faeces and can subsequently be found in litter, soil or contaminated feed. Some strains grow at temperatures as low as 6 °C and thus might be able to replicate in the environment. Infection takes place by the oral route.

Important factors in the pathogenesis of NE are toxin production, composition of feed and interaction with other pathogens.

Death is caused by enterotoxaemia, i.e. by toxins that are produced by *C. perfringens* in the intestines and are absorbed into the bloodstream.

Alpha toxin, which is produced by all types of *C. perfringens*, is a phospholipase which can lyse cell membranes. Purified alpha toxin can kill chickens after oral application, but investigation of field strains showed no correlation between alpha toxin production and NE. However, genetically modified *C. perfringens* not producing alpha toxin were also capable to cause NE (Keyburn et al., 2006). Beta toxin produced by types B and C is poorly characterized but seems to increase capillary permeability (Rainey et al., 2015). Since NE in poultry is mainly caused by types A and C, epsilon and iota toxins produced only by types D are not relevant for the pathogenesis of NE.

Several minor toxins are thought to be involved (Crespo et al., 2007). Of those, pore-forming and cytolytic NetB toxin seems to be the most important toxin (Keyburn et al., 2008). Enterotoxin (CPE) and beta2 toxin (CPB2) were considered as important toxins for enteric diseases but this has been doubted based on epidemiological data (Crespo et al., 2007). Finally, production of bacteriocins by a strain that produces more toxins will allow this strain to replace competing *C. perfringens* strains producing fewer and less toxins (Timbermont et al., 2011).

Feed components that predispose to NE are high protein content as in fishmeal and high content of fibre and complex carbohydrates as a consequence of rations with a high content of the grains wheat, barley or rye. High protein will promote clostridial growth and high fibre will make the ingesta more viscous, slowing down the intestinal passage and promoting clostridial growth, especially in the small intestine. Slower intestinal passage can also be a consequence of skip-a-day feeding, which therefore also predisposes to NE (Opengart and Songer, 2013).

Other intestinal pathogens that damage the intestinal mucosa increase the production of mucus and the release of host protein into the lumen, will further increase clostridial growth and severity of NE. Most important are coccidia including attenuated vaccine strains, but also ascaridia. In turkeys, haemorrhagic enteritis can be associated with NE (Opengart and Songer, 2013).

Clinical signs

4–week-old broilers seem to be most susceptible, but NE has also been described in meat turkeys younger than 9 weeks (Giovanardi et al., 2016).

Birds with NE will often die peracutely without previously showing clinical signs.

If there are symptoms, they are characterized by severe depression, decreased feed consumption and diarrhoea, all of which appear a few hours before death. Mortality increases suddenly and can vary between 1 % and 50 % (Hafez, 2011).

There is also a subclinical form of NE without mortality and symptoms other than reduced weight gain and impaired feed conversion. In spite of the lack of mortality, this form is thought to cause higher economic losses because it will take longer to be diagnosed and subsequently treated (Timbermont et al., 2011).

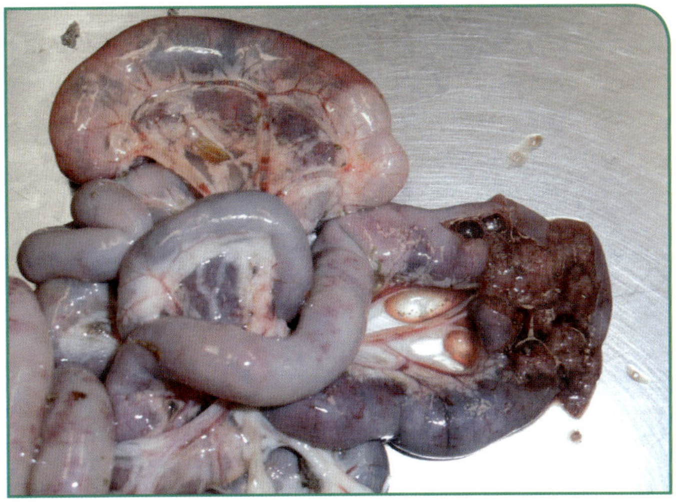

Figure 3. Inflamed and distended intestine.

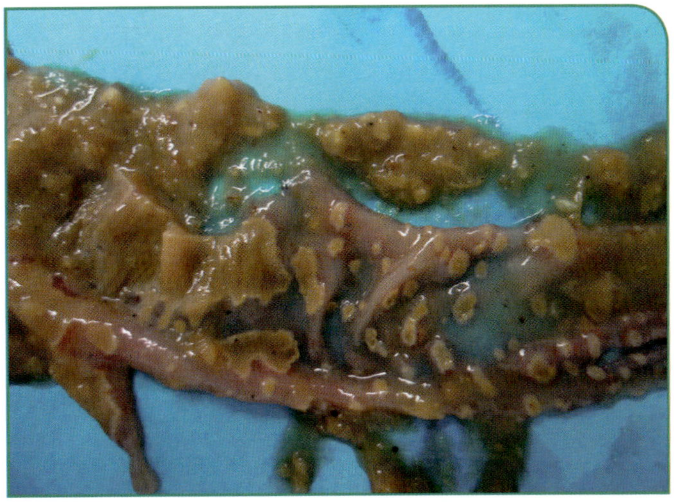

Figure 4. Intestinal mucosa covered with diphteric membrane.

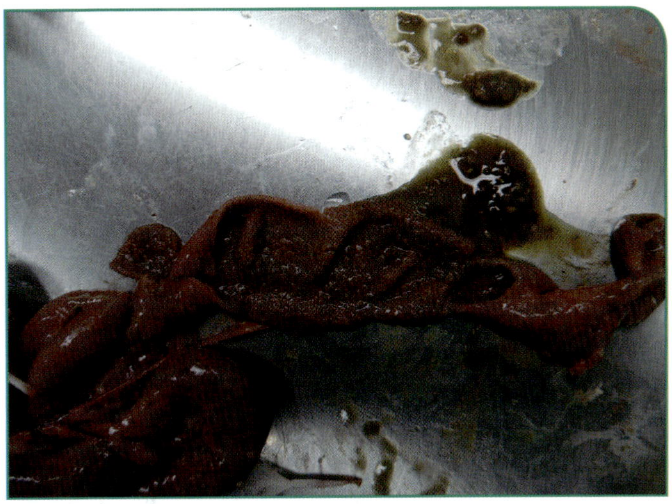

Figure 5. Typical "Turkish towel" appearance.

Post mortem lesions

Gross lesions in birds that have died due to acute NE occur in the jejunum or ileum, rarely in the caeca. The intestines are reddened and/or distended and filled with gas (Fig. 3). Large parts of the intestinal walls are thin and friable and covered by a tightly adherent diphtheric membrane giving the typical "Turkish towel" appearance (Figs. 4 and 5). The content is usually watery or mucous. Microscopically, the lesions are dominated by sloughed off epithelium, coagulation necrosis of the mucosa, which might extend into lower layers of the intestinal wall and is clearly demarked from the healthy tissue. The villi are shortened. Blood vessels are congested and sometimes contain hyaline thrombi. Large numbers of gram-positive rod-shaped bacteria colonize but do not invade the mucosal surface, to which a fibrinous membrane with cellular debris is attached (Fig. 6).

In subclinical cases, lesions are restricted to focal ulcers of the mucosa, which are covered by discoloured and amorphous material. Microscopic lesions are similar as in the acute form, but more inflammatory cells, especially heterophilic granulocytes, are present. Ascending infections with *C. perfringens* can cause liver lesions. In those cases, livers are swollen, paler than usually and show red or white necrotic foci (Fig. 7). Histopathological examination reveals a cholangiohepatitis (Fig. 8).

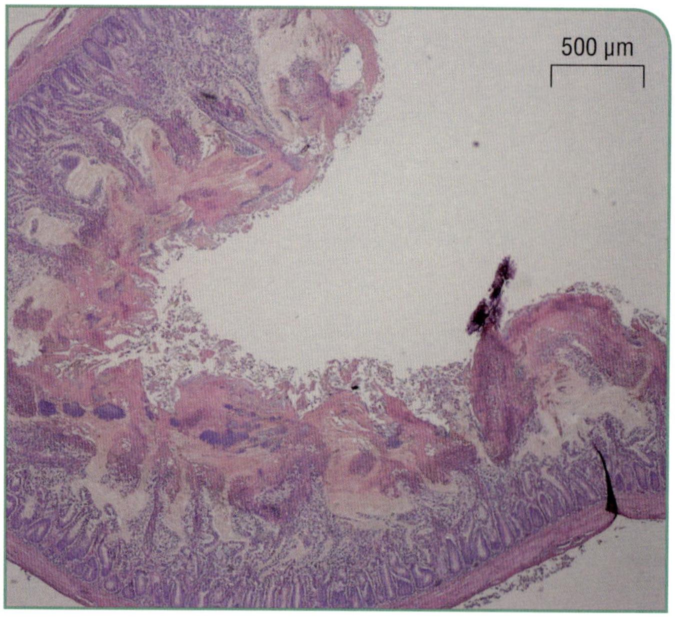

Figure 6. Severe necrotic enteritis: intestinal mucosa covered with diphteric membrane, large bacterial colonies.

Diagnostic procedures

A quick presumptive diagnosis can be made by the detection of abundant numbers of gram-positive, large rods in smears of the necrotic intestinal wall. Spores are not present. *C. perfringens* can readily be isolated from the lesions.

Under anaerobic conditions, the bacterium grows fast on blood agar plates overnight.

Morphology of the colonies can vary, but colonies are usually smooth and glossy and round with a diameter of 2–5 mm. Their colour is grey to yellow. Colonies are surrounded by two zones of haemolysis, an inner smaller with complete haemolysis and an outer wider with incomplete haemolysis (Fig. 9), but the extent and type of haemolysis depends on the production of various haemolysins (Rainey et al., 2015).

Other suitable media are reinforced clostridial medium and egg yolk agar. Reinforced clostridial medium is a non-selective enrichment medium containing peptone, beef extract and yeast extract. Egg yolk agar allows the detection of the lecithinase activity of alpha toxin, which

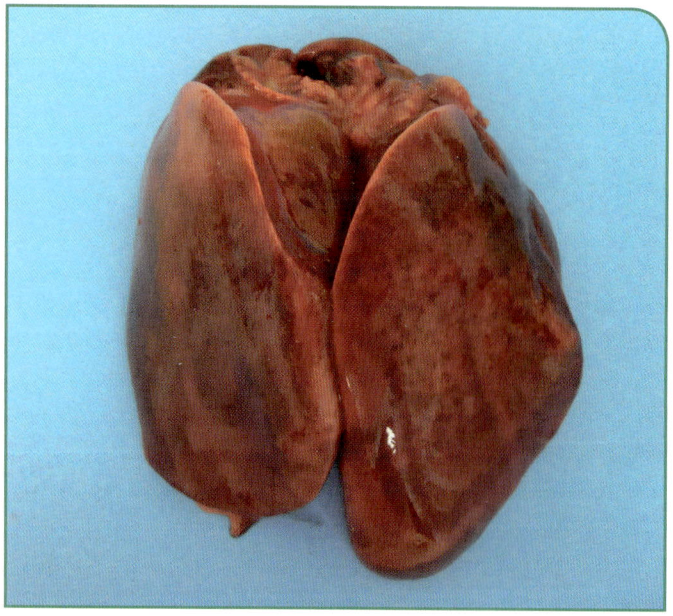

Figure 7. Necrotic foci in the liver due to subclinical necrotic enteritis.

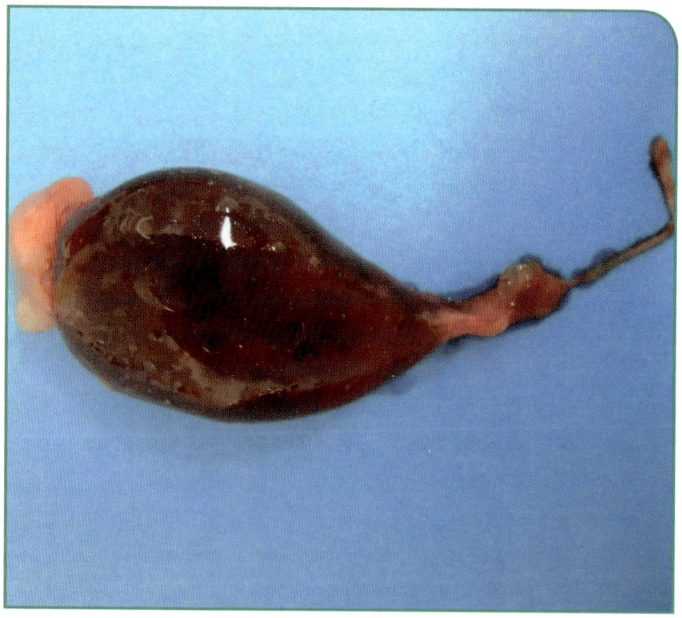

Figure 8. Enlarged gallbladder due to cholangiohepatitis in subclinical necrotic enteritis.

distinguishes *C. perfringens* from most other clostridia. Most isolates ferment lactose, glucose and maltose, hydrolyse gelatine and reduce nitrate. This bacterium is non-motile, indole and catalase negative. The biochemical properties for identification of *C. perfringens* have been described in detail by Rainey et al. (2015).

Because *C. perfringens* can be present in the intestinal flora of healthy chickens, isolation of *C. perfringens* is only diagnostic if it is associated with lesions and present in high numbers of more than 10^5 cfu/g ingesta.

Thus, determination of the bacterial count might be helpful. Tryptose sulphite neomycin (TSN) or tryptose sulphite cycloserine (TSC) agar are probably the most frequently used agar for this purpose. Neomycin or cycloserine inhibit other gram-negative bacteria and some *Clostridia* spp., while *C. perfringens* reduces the sulphite to black ferric sulphide when the plates are incubated at 46 °C (Dafwang et al., 1987).

C. perfringens isolates can be typed using PCRs detecting the toxin genes (Baums et al., 2004). However, the mere presence of genes is not necessarily correlated with virulence. For epidemiological studies, macrorestriction followed by pulsed-field gel electrophoresis (PFGE), sequencing of various toxin genes and multilocus sequence typing (MLST) as well as whole genome sequencing have been used (Lacey et al., 2016). Additionally, ELISAs for direct detection of *C. perfringens* major toxins and enterotoxin are commercially available.

Due to the peracute or acute course of NE and the frequent presence of *C. perfringens* in healthy birds, detection of antibodies against *C. perfringens* is of no diagnostic value.

Treatment

Antibiotics that can be used for the treatment of acute NE include penicillin and other beta-lactamases, tetracyclines, macrolides, bacitracin and virginiamycin. Since resistances of *C. perfringens* against those antibiotics occur, antibacterial susceptibility testing should be done. *C. perfringens* is generally resistant against aminoglycosides (Gad et al., 2011, 2012; Opengart and Songer, 2013). Antibiotics can be given in feed or water. This will decrease further mortality but will not save birds already showing clinical symptoms. To prevent recurrence of the disease after stop of treatment and in cases of subclinical NE, measures listed below should be applied.

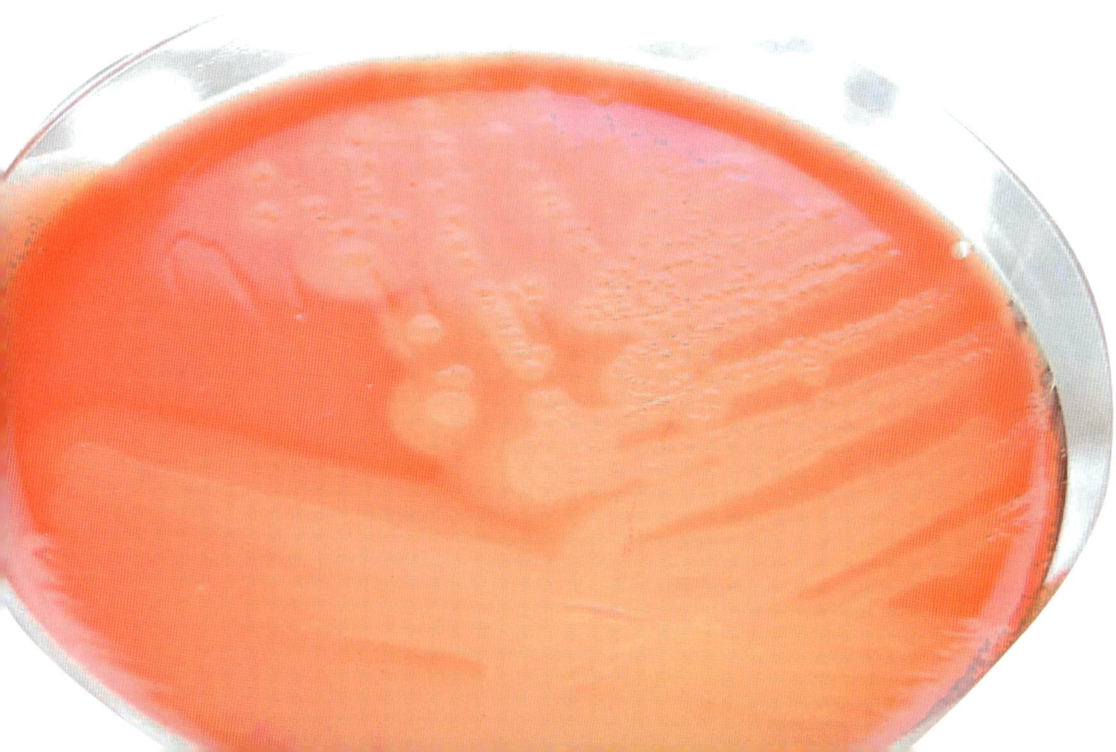

Figure 9. *Clostridium perfringens* colonies on blood agar. Image courtesy of Dr. Sarah Brüggemann-Schwarze (Institute for Poultry Diseases, Freie Universität Berlin).

Control

For a long time, prevention of NE was an effect of the use of antimicrobial growth promoters in the feed, which suppressed the growth of the clostridia and preserved the balance of the intestinal flora. After the ban of their use in the European Union and the trend towards antibiotic-free production in other parts of the world, alternatives are needed.

Most important is to optimize the fee as to avoid predisposing factors such as high protein or fibre content.

Various herbal compounds or organic acids can act directly against *C. perfringens* and reducing their numbers in the intestines. Additionally, a large number of prebiotics and probiotics have been tested for their ability to prevent NE, some of them with success (Caly et al., 2015).

Probiotics are living bacteria or yeasts given in the feed. They can act by interaction with the host, for example by immune modulation. Other probiotics interact with *C. perfringens* by the production of molecules with antimicrobial activities or by outcompeting them otherwise. Examples, which are commercially available, are *Lactobacillus reuteri* or *Saccharomyces cerevisiae* (Caly et al., 2015). Competitive exclusion products, which contain mixed bacterial flora from healthy chickens, can also be effective due to the same mechanisms. Instead of commercial products, it has been claimed that rearing broilers on used litter will help them to establish a normal intestinal flora quicker. Prebiotics support the growth of a balanced intestinal flora. Mostly they are indigestible oligosaccharides like mannan-oligosaccharides (MOS), which are derived from yeast cell walls.

The use of vaccines or bacteriophages against *C. perfringens* has repeatedly been tested; however, no products are commercially available yet.

References

Baums CG, Schotte U, Amtsberg G and Goethe R. Diagnostic multiplex PCR for toxin genotyping of *Clostridium perfringens* isolates. *Veterinary Microbiology*. 2004; 100, 11–16.

Caly DL, D'Inca R, Auclair E and Drider D. Alternatives to antibiotics to prevent necrotic enteritis in broiler chickens: a microbiologist's perspective. *Frontiers in Microbiology*. 2015; 6.

Crespo R, Fisher DJ, Shivaprasad HL, Fernandez-Miyakawa ME and Uzal FA. Toxinotypes of *Clostridium perfringens* isolated from sick and healthy avian species. *Journal of Veterinary Diagnostic Investigation*. 2007; 19, 329–333.

Dafwang II, Ricke SC, Schaefer DM, Brotz PG, Sunde ML and Pringle DJ. Evaluation of some commercial media for the cultivation and enumeration of *Clostridium perfringens* from the chick intestine. *Poultry Science*. 1987; 66, 652–658.

Gad W, Hauck R, Krüger M and Hafez HM. Determination of antibiotic sensitivities of *Clostridium perfringens* isolates from commercial turkeys in Germany in vitro. *Arch. Geflügelk*. 2011; 75, 80–83.

Gad W, Hauck R, Krüger M and Hafez HM. In vitro determination of antibiotic sensitivities of *Clostridium perfringens* isolates from layer flocks in Germany in vitro. *Arch. Geflügelk*. 2012; 76, 234–238.

Giovanardi D, Drigo I, Vidi BD, Agnoletti F, Viel L, Capello K, Berto G and Bano L. Molecular characterization of *Clostridium perfringens* strains isolated from diseased turkeys in Italy. *Avian Pathology*. 2016; 45, 376–380.

Hafez HM. Enteric diseases of poultry with special attention to *Clostridium perfringens*. *Pakistan Veterinary Journal*. 2011; 31, 175–184.

Keyburn AL, Sheedy SA, Ford ME, Williamson MM, Awad MM, Rood JI and Moore RJ. Alpha-toxin of *Clostridium perfringens* is not an essential virulence factor in necrotic enteritis in chickens. *Infection and Immunity*. 2006; 74, 6496–6500.

Keyburn AL, Boyce JD, Vaz P, Bannam TL, Ford ME, Parker D, Di Rubbo A, Rood JI and Moore RJ. NetB, a new toxin that is associated with avian necrotic enteritis caused by *Clostridium perfringens*. *PLoS Pathogens*. 2008; 4, e26.

Labbe RG and Huang TH. Generation times and modeling of enterotoxin-positive and enterotoxin-negative strains of *Clostridium perfringens* in laboratory media and ground beef. *Journal of Food Protection*. 1995; 58, 1303–1306.

Lacey JA, Johanesen PA, Lyras D and Moore RJ. Genomic diversity of necrotic enteritis-associated strains of *Clostridium perfringens*: a review. *Avian Pathology*. 2016; 45, 302–307.

Opengart K and Songer JG. Necrotic enteritis. In: Diseases of Poultry, DE Swayne, JR Glisson, LR McDougald, LK Nolan, DL Suarez and V Nair, eds. Ames, Iowa: Iowa State Press. 2013; pp. 949–953.

Rainey FA, Hollen BJ and Small AM. Clostridium. In: Bergey's Manual of Systematics of Archaea and Bacteria (John Wiley & Sons, Ltd). 2015; DOI: 10.1002/9781118960608.gbm00619.

Songer JG. Clostridia as agents of zoonotic disease. *Veterinary Microbiology*. 2010; 140, 399–404.

Timbermont L, Haesebrouck F, Ducatelle R and Immerseel FV. Necrotic enteritis in broilers: an updated review on the pathogenesis. *Avian Pathology*. 2011; 40, 341–347.

Uzal FA, Sentíes-Cué CG, Rimoldi G and Shivaprasad HL. Non-*Clostridium perfringens* infectious agents producing necrotic enteritis-like lesions in poultry. *Avian Pathology*. 2016; 45, 326–333.

11 Botulism

Botulism is caused by the exotoxins of *Clostridium botulinum*. The disease has also been called "limberneck", describing one of its clinical symptoms. It occurs worldwide and often affects wild waterfowl, especially in warmer weather, when *C. botulinum* thrives in stagnant water, but all types of poultry with or without outdoor access have been affected.

With rare exceptions, botulism of humans and of poultry is caused by different toxin types. However, these exceptions cause some concerns about the risk which outbreaks in poultry may pose for the public health. Flocks with a history of botulism might be slaughtered if they are free of symptoms for several weeks.

Meat from flocks exhibiting clinical signs is not suitable for human consumption.

The decision to slaughter or euthanize a flock should be made after consulting the relevant authorities (Popp et al., 2012).

Aetiology

The name of *C. botulinum* is derived from "botulus", Latin name for little sausage, because canned sausages were a frequent source of botulism. *C. botulinum* is a strictly anaerobe, gram-positive bacterium; its cells are slender, about 4–6 µm long and 1.0 µm wide (Fig. 1). Cells from older cultures undergoing autolysis are gram-variable and can contain oval, subterminal or terminal endospores. *C. botulinum* has peritrichous flagella and is motile. *C. argentinense* is also capable of producing botulinum neurotoxins (BoNT) and causing botulism.

C. botulinum is typed based on cultural properties into four groups, which also comprise closely related *C. sporogenes*, *C. novyi* and *C. subterminale*. However, these *Clostridium* spp. do not produce BoNT, while all *C. botulinum* isolates do. Another typing scheme is based on the BoNT produced. Seven BoNT designated A-G can be distinguished serologically. Almost all cases of botulism in poultry are caused by type C, rarely type D. Types C and D also constitute a cultivar group of their own (Rainey et al., 2015). In recent years, there have been several reports of cases caused by chimeric or mosaic toxin type C/D, parts of which are similar to either type C or type D toxin in Asia and Europe (Skarin et al., 2010; Jang et al., 2014). Besides outbreaks in poultry, toxin type C has caused disease in various mammals like pigs, dogs, horses and cattle. Type C botulism in cattle was caused by feeding chicken manure.

Type C toxin is encoded by phages, which can be lost, turning *C. botulinum* into *C. novyi* (Sakaguchi et al., 2005).

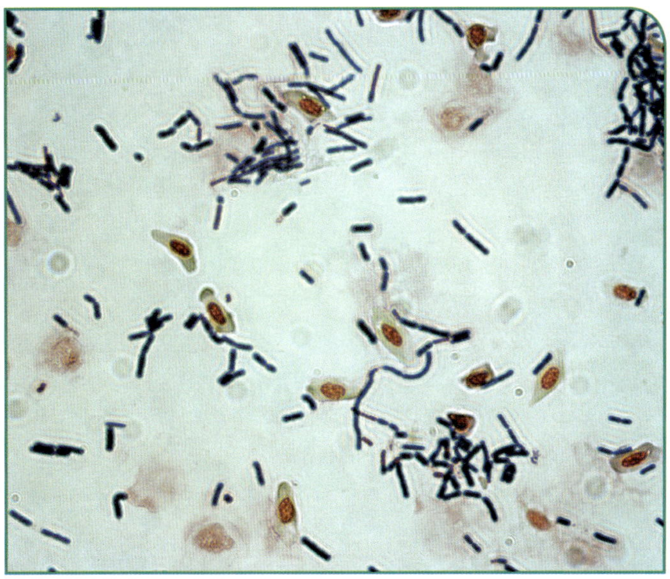

Figure 1. *Clostridium botulinum* cells. Gram stain. Image courtesy of Dr. Sarah Brüggemann-Schwarze (Institute for Poultry Diseases, Freie Universität Berlin).

Pathogenesis and transmission

The symptoms of botulism are caused by BoNT. The toxin is either taken up orally with contaminated feed or produced by *C. botulinum* colonizing the intestines, especially the caeca. The latter condition is called toxicoinfection. *C. botulinum* may be spread by subclinically infected birds shedding the bacterium and its spores in their faeces.

Carcasses in which *C. botulinum* grows and produces its toxin after the death of the host are the most important source of toxin in the environment. This is regardless if the host has died due to botulism or an unrelated condition.

Another source may be invertebrates like maggots feeding on contaminated carcasses or crustaceans in ponds that have died due to a lack of oxygen in warm weather.

BoNTs are considered one of the deadliest poisons with very low minimal lethal doses, so minute amounts of contaminated feed may be sufficient to kill a large number of animals. A single maggot or one gram of a contaminated carcass may contain several thousand minimum lethal doses.

When, as in most cases, no source of the environment can be found in the environment, toxicoinfections are assumed. The concept was proven by reproducing botulism after feeding *C. botulinum* spores, even though some investigations were unable to reproduce those findings. In cases in which experimental toxicoinfection failed, only a low level of BoNT production in the caeca was found. Immunosuppression might facilitate development of the clinical signs after toxicoinfection. The concept of toxicoinfection is further supported by the fact that *C. botulinum* produces more toxin at warmer temperatures encountered inside hosts and at ambient temperatures (Skarin et al., 2013).

BoNT C is produced as an inactive precursor protein, which is cleaved into its active form under slightly alkaline conditions. Compared to other BoNTs, BoNT C is more efficiently absorbed from the intestines. It acts by binding to the presynaptic membrane of neurons followed by uptake in endocytic vesicles and translocation into the cytosol, where it cleaves specific proteins that are necessary for the release of acetylcholine. The inhibition of the release of acetylcholine results in paralysis of the affected muscles.

Clinical signs and post mortem lesions

The time until clinical signs appear after uptake of the toxin as well as the severity of clinical signs are mostly dependent on the dose. Under experimental conditions, the age of the birds was a factor with older birds being more resistant. Under field conditions, age does not seem to play a role (Dohms et al., 1982; Dohms and Cloud, 1982).

In the early stages of the intoxication, birds are reluctant to move and appear lame (Fig. 2). From the legs, flaccid paralysis of the skeletal muscles is progressing cranially, affecting the wings, which droop, the neck and the eyelids (Fig. 3). In the final stage, birds are lying motionless and seemingly dead. Additional signs are feathers that fall out when the birds are handled (Fig. 4) and diarrhoea with large amounts of urates. Death is due to respiratory failure. Cumulative mortalities of up to 40 % in broilers and up to 50 % in turkeys have been reported. Birds can also recover, and within 3 to 4 days paralysis disappears in the reverse order in which it appeared.

There are no gross or histopathological lesions in birds with botulism.

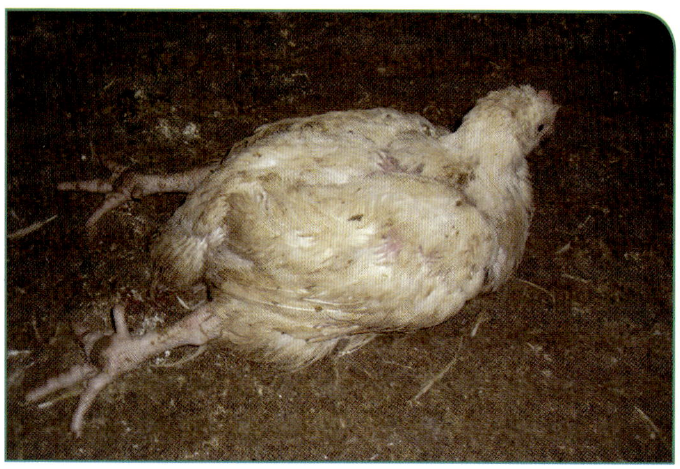

Figure 2. Broiler with paralyzed legs.

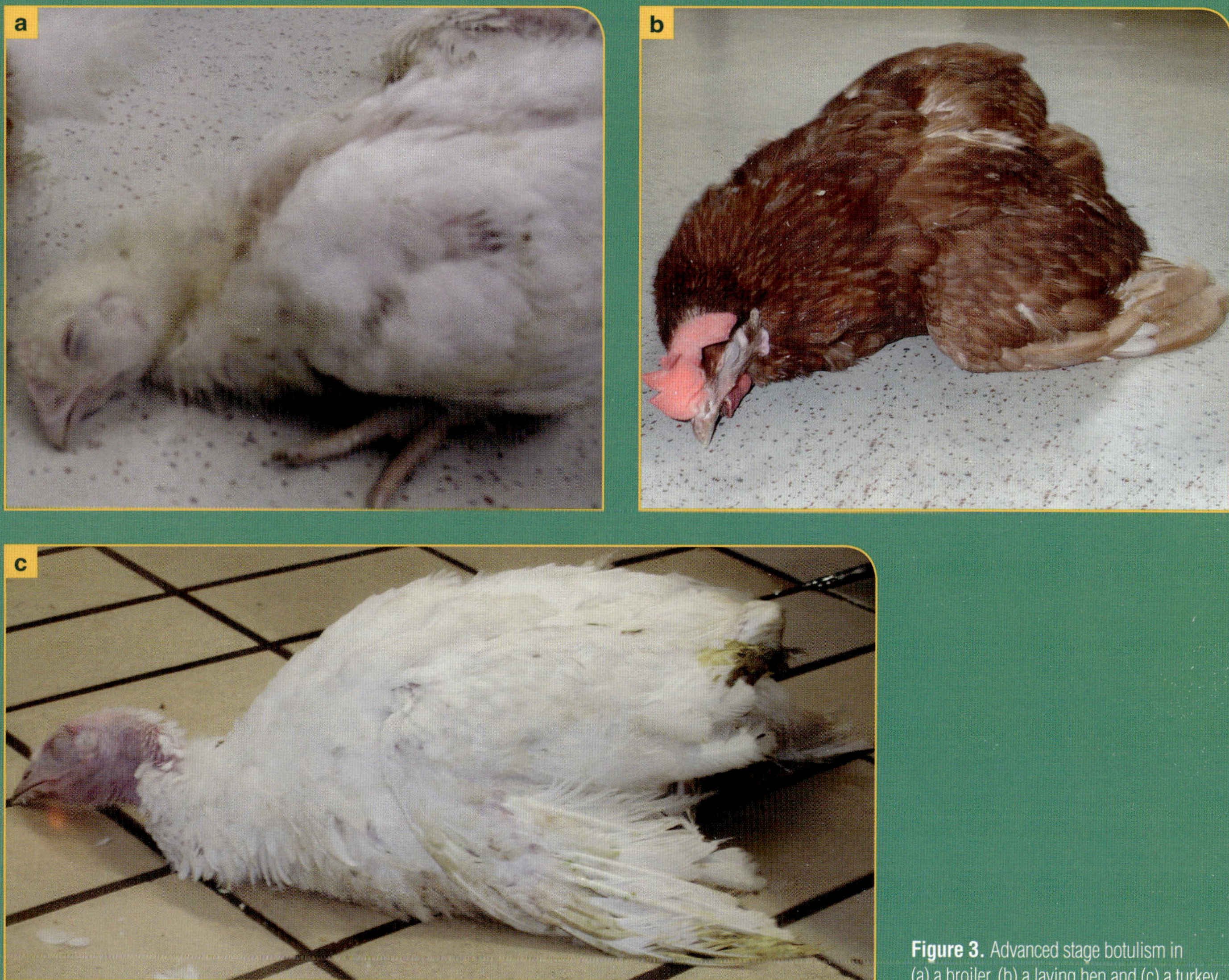

Figure 3. Advanced stage botulism in (a) a broiler, (b) a laying hen and (c) a turkey.

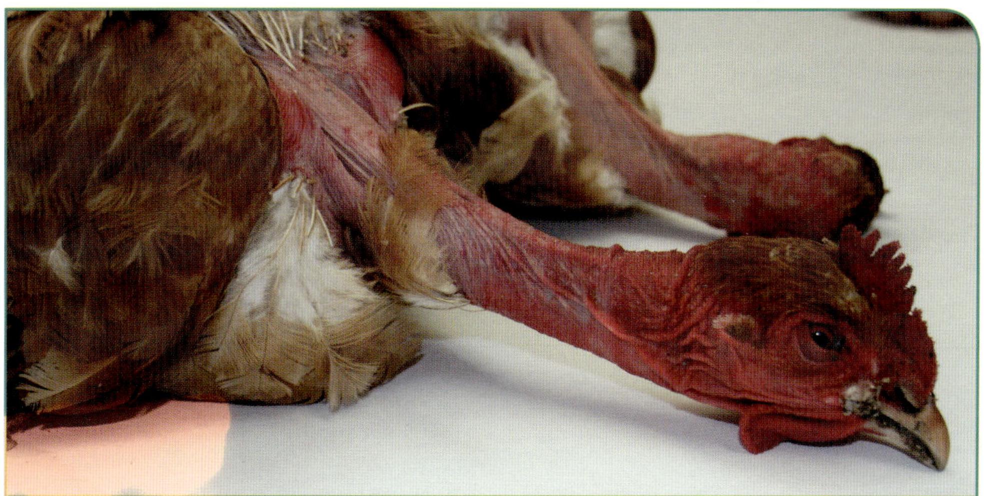

Figure 4. Feather loss due to botulism in hens. Image courtesy of Dr. Bruce Charlton (California Animal Health and Food Safety Laboratory System, Turlock branch).

Diagnostic procedures

The described clinical symptoms in combination with the lack of lesions are very suggestive for botulism and allow a substantiated presumptive diagnosis, but the gold standard of laboratory diagnosis is the detection of BoNT. Suitable samples are serum, liver and to a lesser extent crop or gastrointestinal content. Samples should be taken from euthanized birds showing clinical signs.

The mouse bioassay still is the most widely used method for the detection of BoNTs.

For it, mice are injected intraperitoneally with filtered samples. If the samples contain toxin, the inoculated mice will die showing typical symptoms within a few days. For verification and typing, other mice are inoculated with type-specific antiserum before being given the toxin-containing sample, which will protect them if BoNT and antiserum match. Biological alternatives to using mice are cell-based assays testing receptor binding or function (Eubanks et al., 2007; Basavanna et al., 2013). However, so far these tests have not been evaluated for BoNT C. A variety of antigen capture ELISAs and other immunological methods to detect BoNTs have been described, but most of them are not as sensitive as the mouse bioassay (Grenda et al., 2014). A promising alternative is matrix-assisted laser desorption/ionization – time of flight mass spectrometry (MALDI-TOF MS) assay that detects cleavage of peptide substrates BoNT. Because each BoNT type cleaves a specific substrate, this assay is capable to type the BoNT. The limit of detection was lower than in the mouse bioassay (Boyer et al., 2005).

Isolation of *C. botulinum* from birds or from the environment is of dubious diagnostic value, because the bacterium can be present in birds and flocks without causing disease.

However, in combination with specific clinical signs, the isolation will strengthen the presumptive diagnosis. The most suitable media and temperature depend on the biovar; generally, media rich in protein should be used (Rainey et al., 2015). Enrichment is done in deoxygenated broth medium under anaerobe conditions. Vegetative cells of other bacteria can be inactivated by pasteurizing the broth after addition of the sample, but a not pasteurized sample should also be included (Grenda et al., 2014). After incubation for 3 to 5 days, the supernatant can be tested for BoNT.

On blood agar plates, colonies are grey-white, roundish and 1–5 mm in diameter. A zone of beta-haemolysis surrounds them. The biochemical characteristics of each biovar have been described (Rainey et al., 2015) and molecular methods to genotype *C. botulinum* for epidemiological studies have been reviewed (Grenda et al., 2014).

Treatment

The only aetiological therapy is the parenteral application of type-specific antiserum. This is not a feasible measure in poultry flocks, but has been done with success in individual and valuable birds.

In flocks diagnosed with botulism, the birds should be given the easiest possible access to feed and water. On the other hand, reducing the energy content of the feed might have a beneficial effect in cases caused by toxicoinfections.

Dead birds have to be collected as often as possible, because they are a source of rapid spread of the infection to other birds feeding on them.

Anecdotal evidence suggests that application of sodium selenite and vitamins A, D_3 and E might reduce mortality. Furthermore, treatment with antibiotics seemed to be effective in some but not all cases (Skarin et al., 2013). *C. botulinum* is generally susceptible to macrolides, betalactamases and tetracyclines; it is resistant to gentamicin (Rainey et al., 2015).

Control

Prompt removal of organic matter and especially dead animals that might harbour *C. botulinum* will help to prevent outbreaks. However, the spores are difficult to disinfect. Calcium hypochlorite, iodophors and formalin have been recommended for this purpose (Skarin et al., 2013).

A different approach is to inhibit the growth of *C. botulinum* in the intestinal tract, for example by adding citric acid to the drinking water or avoiding excessively high iron content of the water. It is unknown if other measures to establish and maintain a healthy intestinal flora might have any influence on toxicoinfections.

Toxoid vaccines against BoNT C are available in some countries, but they are only licensed for other animals like cattle or mink and not for poultry. Under experimental conditions and in broilers on farms with a history of botulism were effective. A booster vaccine 2 weeks after a first application is recommended (Anniballi et al., 2013).

References

Anniballi F, Fiore A, Löfström C, Skarin H, Auricchio B, Woudstra C, Bano L, Segerman B, Koene M and Båverud V. Management of animal botulism outbreaks: from clinical suspicion to practical countermeasures to prevent or minimize outbreaks. *Biosecurity and Bioterrorism: Biodefense Strategy, Practice and Science.* 2013; 11 S1, 91–S199.

Basavanna U, Muruvanda T, Brown EW and Sharma SK. Development of a cell-based functional assay for the detection of *Clostridium botulinum* neurotoxin types A and E. *International Journal of Microbiology.* 2013; e593219.

Boyer AE, Moura H, Woolfitt AR, Kalb SR, McWilliams LG, Pavlopoulos A, Schmidt JG, Ashley DL and Barr JR. From the mouse to the mass spectrometer: detection and differentiation of the endoproteinase activities of botulinum neurotoxins a–g by mass spectrometry. *Analytical Chemistry.* 2005; 77, 3916–3924.

Dohms JE and Cloud SS. Susceptibility of broiler chickens to *Clostridium botulinum* type C toxin. *Avian Diseases.* 1982; 26, 89–96.

Dohms JE, Allen PH and Rosenberger JK. Cases of type C botulism in broiler chickens. *Avian Diseases.* 1982; 26, 204–210.

Eubanks LM, Hixon MS, Jin W, Hong S, Clancy CM, Tepp WH, Baldwin MR, Malizio CJ, Goodnough MC, Barbieri JT, Johnson EA, Boger DL, Dickerson TJ and Janda KD. An in vitro and in vivo disconnect uncovered through high-throughput identification of botulinum neurotoxin A antagonists. *Proceedings of the National Academy of Sciences.* 2007; 104, 2602–2607.

Grenda T, Kukier E and Kwiatek K. Methods and difficulties in detection of *Clostridium botulinum* and its toxins. *Polish Journal of Veterinary Sciences.* 2014; 17, 195–205.

Jang I, Kang M-S, Kim H-R, Oh J, Lee J-I, Lee H-S and Kwon Y-K. Occurrence of avian botulism in Korea during the period from june to september 2012. *Avian Diseases.* 2014; 58, 666–669.

Popp C, Hauck R, Gad W and Hafez HM. Type C botulism in a commercial turkey farm: a case report. *Avian Diseases.* 2012; 56, 760–763.

Rainey FA, Hollen BJ and Small AM. Clostridium. In: Bergey's Manual of Systematics of Archaea and Bacteria (John Wiley & Sons, Ltd). 2015; DOI: 10.1002/9781118960608.gbm00619.

Sakaguchi Y, Hayashi T, Kurokawa K, Nakayama K, Oshima K, Fujinaga Y, Ohnishi M, Ohtsubo E, Hattori M and Oguma K. The genome sequence of *Clostridium botulinum* type C neurotoxin-converting phage and the molecular mechanisms of unstable lysogeny. *Proceedings of the National Academy of Sciences.* U.S.A. 2005; 102, 17472–17477.

Skarin H, Lindberg A, Blomqvist G, Aspán A and Båverud V. Molecular characterization and comparison of *Clostridium botulinum* type C avian strains. *Avian Pathology.* 2010; 39, 511–518.

Skarin H, Blomqvist G and Båverud V. Botulism. In: Diseases of Poultry, DE Swayne, JR Glisson, LR McDougald, LK Nolan, DL Suarez and V Nair, eds. Ames, Iowa: Iowa State Press. 2013; pp. 953–957.

12 Erysipelas

Erysipelothrix rhusiopathiae is the causing agent of erysipelas, a sporadically but worldwide occurring infection of many vertebrate species. The disease is most significant in swine; in birds, it is mostly regarded as a disease of turkeys, but it can also be a problem in chickens, ducks, geese, pheasants and quail.

Erysipelas usually takes an acute septicaemic course; chronic inflammations localized in joints or at the cardiac valves occur less often.

Economic damage results from mortality, lost productivity, drop in egg production and condemnation at slaughter due to signs of septicaemia.

In humans, the disease caused by *E. rhusiopathiae* is called erysipeloid, while the disease called erysipelas is caused by *Streptococcus* spp. In most cases, erysipeloid is a mild and self-limiting inflammation of the skin characterized by a well marked off, slightly elevated, purple area. In more severe cases, it can spread to other sites of the skin, to adjacent joints and to other organs causing systemic disease with septicaemia. Erysipeloid is considered an occupational disease, since it is acquired through infection of skin wounds when handling infected animals, most importantly fish. There is no known transmission between humans.

Aetiology

The genus *Erysipelothrix* is placed into the class Erysipelotrichia. Erysipelotrichia are closely related to the Bacilli, which include *Lactobacilli* and *Listeria*, and Clostridia (Stackebrandt, 2015). *Erysipelothrix* spp. stain gram-positive but are gram-labile. Usually, they are slender rods, measuring 0.2–0.4 by 0.8-2.5 µm and may be slightly curved. After several passages the cells may look more filamentous (Fig. 1). *E. rhusiopathiae* does not form spores; it is anaerobic and catalase-negative.

The other species in the genus is *E. tonsillarum*, which was split off from *E. rhusiopathiae* based on DNA-hybridization results and its ability to produce acid from saccharose (Takahashi et al., 1992). Because they were historically regarded as one species, *E. rhusiopathiae* and *E. tonsillarum* share the same serotyping system (Kucsera, 1973). A total of 26 serotypes have been described and are designated 1a, 1b, 2a, 2b, 3 – 23 or N, whereas N designates isolates lacking the type-specific antigen. Seven serotypes (3, 7, 10, 14, 20, 22 and 23) are *E. tonsillarum*; the others are *E. rhusiopathiae*. *E. tonsillarum* is considered to be apathogenic for chickens. Investigations of serotyping poultry isolates are very rare. Isolates from laying hens mainly belonged to serovars 1a, 1b, 2b, 4, 5, 6 or 11, while isolates from turkeys belonged to serovars 1b, 2 or 5.

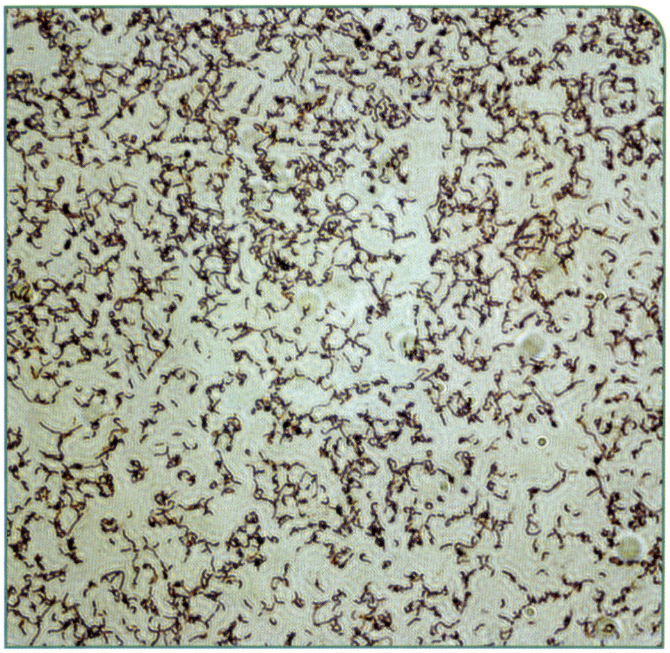

Figure 1. *Erysipelothrix rhusiopathiae* cells. Gram stain. Image courtesy of Dr. Sarah Brüggemann-Schwarze (Institute for Poultry Diseases, Freie Universität Berlin).

It has been repeatedly suggested that *E. rhusiopathiae* can multiply in soil under favourable conditions. However, controlled experiments showed that, under optimal cool and moist conditions with low organic matter, *E. rhusiopathiae* can stay infective only for up to 5 weeks in soil (Wood, 1973). The bacteria are very resistant in meat or other tissues, in which they can survive smoking, pickling, freezing and decay. However, it is not very resistant against common disinfectants (Bricker and Saif, 2013).

Pathogenesis and transmission

Infections with *E. rhusiopathiae* often take place by direct or indirect contact with other infected animals. Since the host spectrum comprises many mammals, birds, reptiles, amphibians and fish, there is a long list of potential living vectors (Bricker and Saif, 2013). In practice, probably rodents are most relevant. Pigs and sheep can often be easily and subclinically infected with *E. rhusiopathiae*, and poultry can acquire the infection from them, either by using pens previously occupied by infected pigs or sheep or by indirect contact via fomites. *E. rhusiopathiae* has often been associated with fish, but also molluscs and crustaceans. While direct or indirect contact of poultry with fish might be rare, improperly prepared fishmeal can be a source of infection. *E. rhusiopathiae* has also been repeatedly isolated from the red fowl mite, which can serve as mechanical vector, as probably biting insects do. The bacteria frequently survive in the outdoor environment or in poultry houses after inadequate cleaning and disinfection. They then can infect the next flock.

The main route of infection is via skin wounds. Thus, fighting between turkey toms, artificial insemination of turkey hens or toe trimming of young poults are potential risk factors because they can cause skin injuries.

Oral infection can be successful under experimental conditions, but it is thought that in these cases small wounds in the mucosa are the actual portals of entry. Cannibalism on birds that succumbed to the disease will also transmit the infection. The possibility of vertical transmission of erysipelas has been excluded (Mazaheri et al., 2006).

From the site of infection, *E. rhusiopathiae* spreads in the blood, causing septicaemia and/or infecting some organs. It is facultative intracellular in macrophages. The bacteria are shed in the faeces. Persistent infection and carrier status can occur in turkeys and seems to be more frequent in chickens (Nakazawa et al., 1998).

Isolates of *E. rhusiopathiae* can differ in their virulence regardless of their serotype, and a number of virulence factors are known. These include the enzymes coagulase, which might help to produce a protective layer around the bacterial cells, and neuraminidase, which is involved in entry into host cells. Adhesins and presence of a capsule are also important for attachment; the capsule also increases resistance to phagocytosis. Survival in macrophages after phagocytosis may be facilitated by antioxidant factors, stress proteins and phospholipases (Shimoji, 2000). Full genome sequencing yielded more genes potentially related to virulence (Ogawa et al., 2011). *E. rhusiopathiae* produces no known toxins.

Clinical signs

The incubation period is between 1 to 5 days. Birds may die peracutely without having displayed clinical signs or first show non-specific symptoms like general weakness with unsteady gait, ruffled feathers and a drop in egg production in laying turkey hens and laying hens of up to 70 %. More specific signs are diarrhoea, purple and swollen skin lesions, especially at the snood of toms (Fig. 2), and emaciation in chronic cases.

Birds with clinical signs will almost certainly succumb to the disease, so that morbidity and mortality are almost identical and will continue until a flock is slaughtered if left untreated.

Morbidity and mortality depend mostly on the virulence of the strain and the host species, with turkeys being more susceptible than chickens. Under experimental conditions in specific pathogen-free (SPF) chickens, infection by the oral route causes less morbidity and mortality than intramuscular application. In turkeys, age and sex are not regarded a determining factor. In chickens, it is suspicious that erysipelas is almost exclusively a disease of laying hens and not of broilers or pullets. Older hens seem to be more susceptible (Mazaheri et al., 2005). Depending on these factors, mortality can vary considerably. Daily mortality is low but cumulative mortality may be up to 50 % in chickens and turkeys.

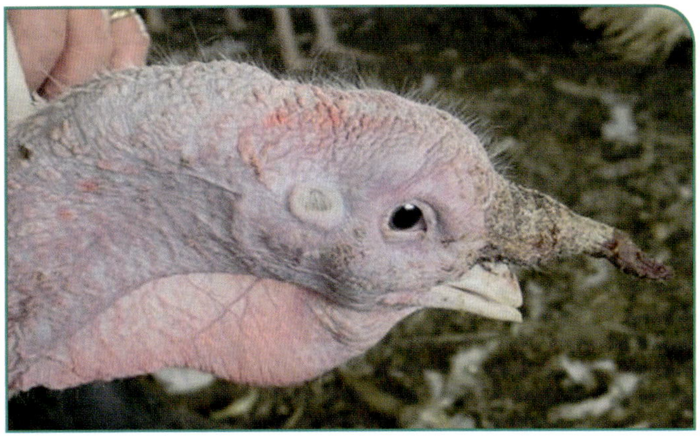

Figure 2. Swollen snood.

Post mortem lesions

Gross lesions are similar in all species and indicate septicaemia. They are characterized by congested blood vessels in the internal organs, dark muscles as well as by petechial haemorrhages in the heart muscle (Fig. 3) and in pericardial and abdominal fat. The parenchymatous organs such as liver and spleen are enlarged, friable and mottled due to necrotic areas (Figs. 4 and 5). Peritonitis and pericarditis may be present. Catarrhal enteritis is frequently observed and small yellow nodules in the caeca have been described. Other organs that are frequently inflamed are the oviduct, especially after infection during artificial insemination, joints and the endocardium (Fig. 6). The ovary can be regressed and discoloured.

Main histopathological lesions are congested blood vessels in all organs. Intravascular coagulation with bacterial nests is frequent and hyalinization of the walls can be observed. Oedema and haemorrhages are a consequence.

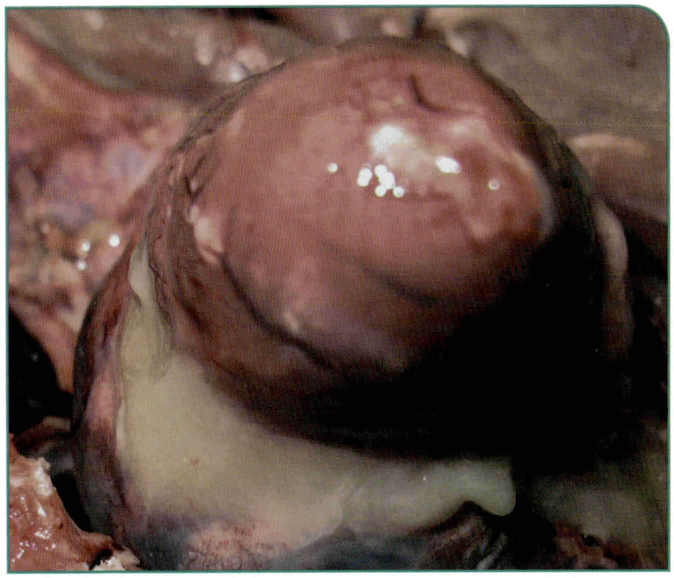

Figure 3. Haemorrhages in the heart muscle.

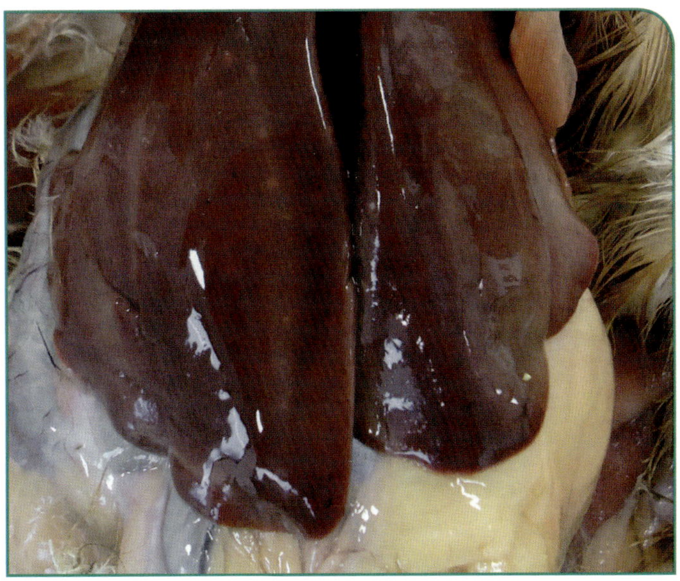

Figure 4. Swollen liver with necrotic foci.

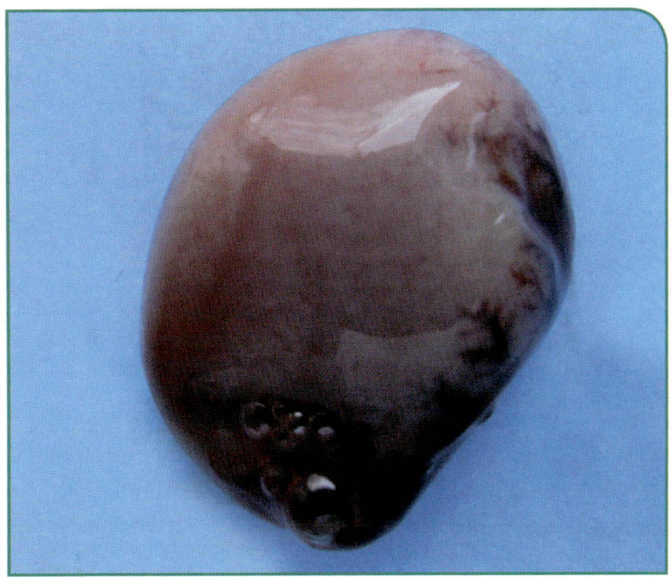

Figure 5. Swollen spleen with necrosis.

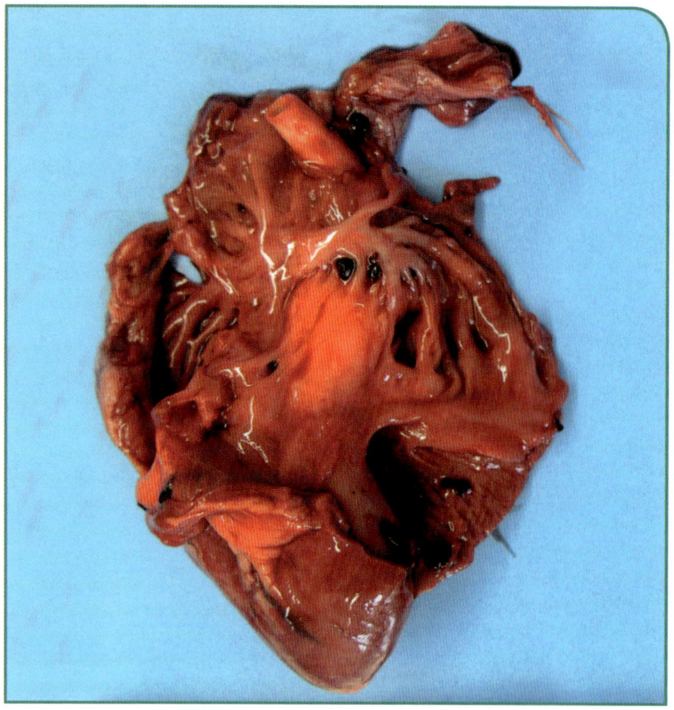

Figure 6. Endocarditis.

In the liver, degeneration of hepatocytes and sometimes areas of necrosis are present. Kupffer cells contain bacteria. Lesions in the spleen are severe loss of lymphocytes, hyalinization of sheathed arteries, necrosis and macrophages containing bacteria. Degenerative lesions can also be observed in the kidney and to a lesser extent in other organs like lung, heart and gastrointestinal tract. Inflammation in affected organs is characterized by fibrin deposition; infiltration of inflammatory cells may be almost lacking in acute cases, but may be present if the disease takes a protracted course.

Diagnostic procedures

If septicaemia is suspected based on the gross lesions, detection of gram-positive slender bacteria in blood smears or organ smears of liver, spleen or bone marrow will point to *E. rhusiopathiae*.

Samples for isolation of the bacterium should be taken from birds that died, since they will have a higher bacterial load compared to culled birds. Liver, spleen and bone marrow are preferred samples.

Selective media containing sodium azide-crystal violet or a combination of antibiotics have been described (Packer, 1943; Wood, 1965). However, they can also inhibit the growth of some *E. rhusiopathiae* strains, so samples should be cultured additionally on blood agar (Fig. 7). Plates should be incubated at 37 °C microaerophilicly or in an atmosphere containing 5–10 % CO_2.

Colonies are about 0.5–0.8 mm in diameter, smooth and dewy; in rare cases or after several passages, they are rough, opaque, dry and 1–2 mm in diameter. Colonies frequently have a small zone of alpha haemolysis. Most important biochemical characteristics are gelatinase activity indicated by brush type of growth in gelatine stab culture incubated at 21 °C and H_2S production as indicated by blackened lead acetate agar or triple-sugar iron (TSI) agar or Kligler's agar. Serotyping is done using heat-stable antigen extracts by tube agglutination of agar gel precipitation test (Wellmann et al., 1983).

Several PCR assays for identification of *E. rhusiopathiae* and differentiation from *E. tonsillarum* from culture or its detection in samples have been validated and published, e.g. by Yamazaki et al. (2006).

Molecular biological methods used for strain differentiation in epidemiological studies included, amongst others, randomly amplified polymorphic DNA methods, macrorestriction enzyme analysis followed by pulsed-field gel electrophoresis (PFGE), multilocus sequence typing (MLST) and sequencing the hypervariable region of the surface protective antigen (SpaA) gene (Janßen et al., 2015).

Detection of antibodies is usually not regarded a helpful tool in diagnosis of acute erysipelas, but has been used to screen chicken flocks for exposure. For that purpose, an ELISA designed for detection of antibodies in pigs was modified and validated (Kurian et al., 2012). Other tests used in swine include various agglutination tests.

Treatment

The universally recommended antibiotic to reduce morbidity and mortality in case of an outbreak is penicillin. Treatment should start as soon as possible by intramuscular application of a rapid acting formulation, because birds already showing symptoms will not consume medicated feed or water. After the initial treatment, a switch to peroral application is possible. When the treatment is stopped, the disease will flare up again, because the bacterium persists in the environment and in carriers. To prevent that, diseased flocks should be vaccinated with bacterins (Bricker and Saif, 2013).

Due to the usually good success of treatment with penicillin, investigations about antimicrobial susceptibility of *E. rhusiopathiae* are rare.

Screening of isolates from various hosts showed a good susceptibility against various antibiotics with the exception of tetracyclines, but confirmed that penicillin had the lowest minimal inhibitory concentrations (MICs) (Fidalgo et al., 2002).

Control

The control of erysipelas relies on prevention of introduction of *E. rhusiopathiae* into flocks and on vaccination. Due to the wide host spectrum and relatively high tenacity of the bacterium, it is difficult to reliably prevent the introduction into flocks with outdoor access. However, routine hygiene measures like cleaning and disinfection of equipment and pest control will help if done thoroughly. In case of outbreaks, it is important to remove dead birds as soon as possible, since they are an important source of infection.

Inactivated as well as live vaccines for turkeys are available in some countries. They should be used in flocks neighbouring or following an infected flock and generally where erysipelas is a common problem.

Bacterin vaccines contain a mixture of serotypes 1 and 2; the protection offered by them is serotype specific. In contrast, attenuated live vaccines induce cross-protection in swine (Redhead et al., 1998). Meat turkeys can be vaccinated with bacterins once, while for breeder turkeys a booster vaccination after 4 weeks is recommended. Live vaccines always require a booster vaccination. In countries without registered vaccines against *E. rhusiopathiae*, autogenous vaccines should be used. Vaccines for pigs should not be used off label, since they are not always protective for turkeys, even if they contain the right serotypes. Furthermore, there might be legal obstacles in some jurisdictions.

There is only limited experience in chickens. In at least one instance, the use of a vaccine for pigs was not successful (Hafez et al., 2001).

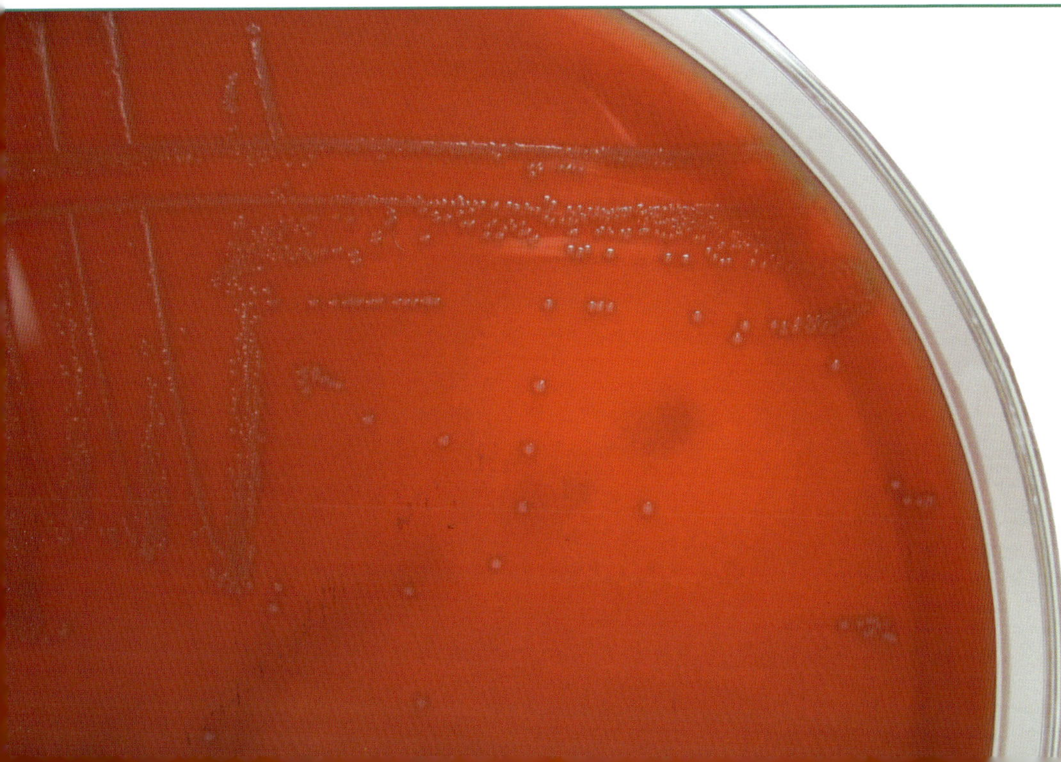

Figure 7. *Erysipelothrix rhusiopathiae* colonies on blood agar. Image courtesy of Dr. Sarah Brüggemann-Schwarze (Institute for Poultry Diseases, Freie Universität Berlin).

References

BRICKER JM AND SAIF YM. Erysipelas. In: Diseases of Poultry, DE Swayne, JR Glisson, LR McDougald, LK Nolan, DL Suarez and V Nair, eds. Ames, Iowa: Iowa State Press. 2013; pp. 986–994.

FIDALGO SG, LONGBOTTOM CJ AND RILEY TV. Susceptibility of *Erysipelothrix rhusiopathiae* to antimicrobial agents and home disinfectants. *Pathology (Philadelphia, Pa.)*. 2002; 34, 462–465.

HAFEZ HM, MAZAHERI A, PRUSAS C, BÖHLAND K, PÖPPEL M AND SCHULZE D. Aktuelle Geflügelkrankheiten bei Legehennen im Zusammenhang mit alternativen Haltungssystemen. *Tierärztliche Praxis*. 2001; 29 (G), 168–174.

JANSSEN T, VOSS M, KÜHL M, SEMMLER T, PHILIPP H-C AND EWERS C. A combinational approach of multilocus sequence typing and other molecular typing methods in unravelling the epidemiology of *Erysipelothrix rhusiopathiae* strains from poultry and mammals. *Veterinary Research*. 2015; 46, 84.

KUCSERA G. Proposal for standardization of the designations used for serotypes of Erysipelothrix rhusiopathiae (Migula) Buchanan. *International Journal of Systematic and Evolutionary Microbiology*. 1973; 23, 184–188.

KURIAN A, NEUMANN EJ, HALL WF AND CHRISTENSEN N. Development of an enzyme-linked immunosorbent assay for the serological detection of exposure of poultry in New Zealand to *Erysipelothrix rhusiopathiae* and their serological response to vaccination. *New Zealand Veterinary Journal*. 2012; 60, 100–105.

MAZAHERI A, LIERZ M AND HAFEZ HM. Investigations on the pathogenicity of *Erysipelothrix rhusiopathiae* in laying hens. *Avian Diseases*. 2005; 49, 574–576.

MAZAHERI A, PHILIPP HC, BONSACK H AND VOSS M. Investigations of the vertical transmission of *Erysipelothrix rhusiopathiae* in laying hens. *Avian Diseases*. 2006; 50, 306–308.

NAKAZAWA H, HAYASHIDANI H, HIGASHI J, KANEKO K, TAKAHASHI T AND OGAWA M. Occurrence of *Erysipelothrix* spp. in broiler chickens at an abattoir. *Journal of Food Protection*. 1998; 61, 907–909.

OGAWA Y, OOKA T, SHI F, OGURA Y, NAKAYAMA K, HAYASHI T AND SHIMOJI Y. The genome of *Erysipelothrix rhusiopathiae*, the causative agent of swine erysipelas, reveals new insights into the evolution of firmicutes and the organism's intracellular adaptations. *Journal of Bacteriology*. 2011; 193, 2959–2971.

PACKER RA. The use of sodium azide (NaN3) and crystal violet in a selective medium for Streptococci and *Erysipelothrix rhusiopathiae*. *Journal of Bacteriology*. 1943; 46, 343–349.

REDHEAD K, PUGH CA, JENSEN NE AND HOUGHTON SB. Cross protection against *Erysipelothrix rhusiopathiae* serotype 10 induced by a serotype 1 and 2 vaccine. *Veterinary Record*. 1998; 142, 612.

SHIMOJI Y. Pathogenicity of *Erysipelothrix rhusiopathiae*: virulence factors and protective immunity. *Microbes and Infection*. 2000; 2, 965–972.

STACKEBRANDT E. Erysipelothrix. In: Bergey's Manual of Systematics of Archaea and Bacteria (John Wiley & Sons, Ltd). 2015; DOI: 10.1002/9781118960608.fbm00153.

TAKAHASHI T, FUJISAWA T, TAMURA Y, SUZUKI S, MURAMATSU M, SAWADA T, BENNO Y AND MITSUOKA T. DNA relatedness among *Erysipelothrix rhusiopathiae* strains representing all twenty-three serovars and *Erysipelothrix tonsillarum*. *International Journal of Systematic Bacteriology*. 1992; 42, 469–473.

WELLMANN G, KUCSERA G AND NORRUNG V. Comparative studies on different methods in typing strains of *Erysipelothrix-rhusiopathiae*. 1. Methods and influence of some factors. *Zentralblatt Bakteriol. Mikrobiol. Hyg. Ser. -Med. Microbiol. Infect. Dis. Virol. Parasitol.* 1983; 254, 42–54.

WOOD R. A selective liquid medium utilizing antibiotics for isolation of *Erysipelothrix insidiosa*. *American Journal of Veterinary Research*. 1965; 26, 1303–1308.

WOOD R. Survival of *Erysipelothrix rhusiopathiae* in soil under various environmental conditions. *Cornell Veterinarian*. 1973; 63, 390–410.

YAMAZAKI Y. A multiplex polymerase chain reaction for discriminating *Erysipelothrix rhusiopathiae* from *Erysipelothrix tonsillarum*. *Journal of Veterinary Diagnostic Investigation*. 2006; 18, 384–387.

13 Infections with gram-positive cocci

Gram-positive cocci causing disease in poultry are *Staphylococcus aureus*, *Streptococcus* spp. and *Enterococcus* spp. They are worldwide commonly occurring bacteria that are often isolated from diseased chickens and turkeys. They are frequently associated with localized lesions in the musculoskeletal system and sometimes with lesions in other organs. They are also capable to cause septicaemia.

Green-liver disease or green-liver osteomyelitis complex is a syndrome in turkeys mostly associated with *Staph. aureus*, among other bacteria. By causing these lesions, gram-positive cocci lead to impaired production parameters including increased condemnation rates at slaughter.

In addition to chickens and turkeys, gram-positive cocci can infect other bird species and mammals including humans, where, as in poultry, they can cause wound infections and/or septicaemia.

Methicillin-resistant *Staph. aureus* (MRSA), which are resistant against practically all beta-lactam antibiotics, and vancomycin-resistant enterococci (VRE) are regarded as a major public health problem and can be found in poultry.

Furthermore, *Staph. aureus* isolates producing enterotoxins can cause food poisoning. Such *Staph. aureus* isolates derived either from workers or from the slaughtered birds can contaminate carcasses at slaughter.

On the other hand, enterococci are also used as probiotics in humans and poultry (Franz et al., 2011; Caly et al., 2015).

Aetiology

Staph. aureus, *Streptococcus* spp. and *Enterococcus* spp. are immobile, non-spore-forming, facultative anaerobic, gram-positive staining, coccoid bacteria. All of them belong to the class Bacilli; within this, the genus *Staphylococcus* belongs to the order Bacillales, while *Streptococcus* spp. and *Enterococcus* spp. belong to different families of the order Lactobacillales.

More practically relevant is that *Staphylococcus* spp. are usually positive in the catalase reaction, and their cells occur in clusters when grown on solid media (Fig. 1). In contrast, *Streptococcus* spp. and *Enterococcus* spp. are usually negative in the catalase reaction, and their cells occur in chains (Fig. 2) (Andreasen, 2013; Thayer and Waltman, 2013).

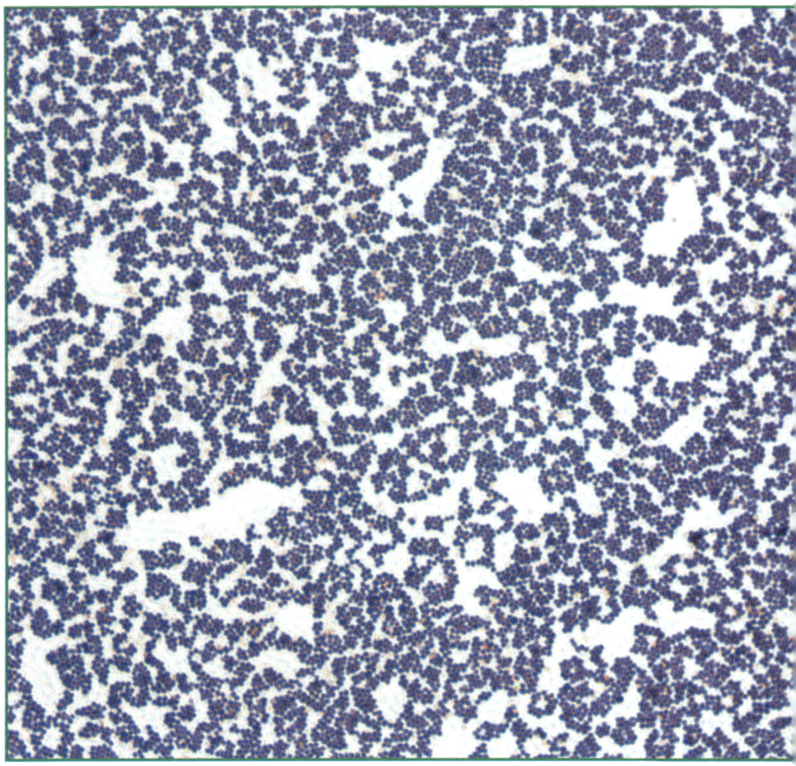

Figure 1. *Staphylococcus aureus* cells. Gram stain. Image courtesy of Dr. Sarah Brüggemann-Schwarze (Institute for Poultry Diseases, Freie Universität Berlin).

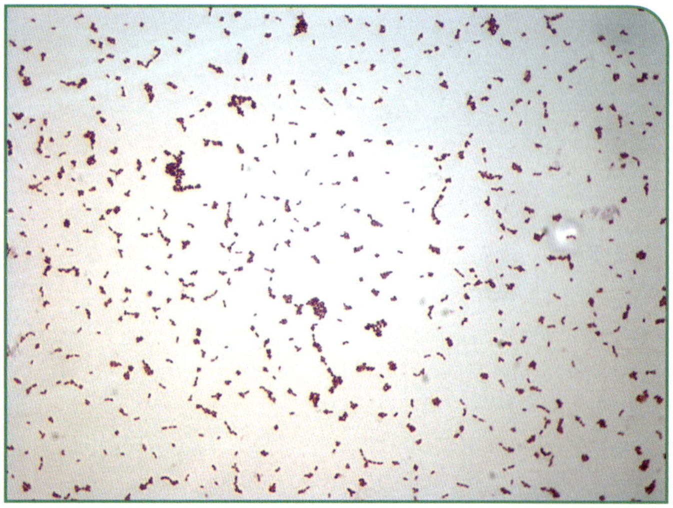

Figure 2. *Streptococcus mutans* cells. Gram stain. Image courtesy of Dr. Sarah Brüggemann-Schwarze (Institute for Poultry Diseases, Freie Universität Berlin).

Pathogenesis and transmission

Staph. aureus, *Streptococcus* spp. and *Enterococcus* spp. are ubiquitous bacteria and opportunistic pathogens. *Staph. aureus* is part of the normal bacterial flora of the skin, while, as their name suggests, *Enterococcus* spp. can be part of the normal intestinal flora. *Streptococcus* spp. reside on the skin as well as in the intestines. Transmission of virulent *Str. zooepidemicus* from horses to chickens has been shown (Bisgaard et al., 2012).

Infection leading to disease with *Staph. aureus* happens mostly through skin wounds or through the open navel after hatch, while *Streptococcus* spp. and *Enterococcus* spp. cause lesions mainly after oral or aerosol infection.

Staph. aureus is the only member of its genus that is pathogenic for poultry, even though *Staph. hyicus* was occasionally found to be associated with lesions. It should be noted that, in spite of its name, *Staph. gallinarum* is avirulent for poultry, but is an opportunistic human bacterial pathogen (Shi et al., 2015).

Catalase-negative, gram-positive cocci have historically been divided into Lancefield groups based on their serological properties, but the typing scheme has lost relevance in recent decades. Most of the Lancefield groups belong to the genus *Streptococcus*, while Lancefield groups D and E constitute the genus *Enterococcus*.

Streptococcus spp. that have been found to be associated with disease in poultry are mostly *Str. equi* subsp. *zooepidemicus* and *Str. gallolyticus*. They further include lesser-known species like *Str. gallinaceus* or *Str. pluranimalium* (Thayer and Waltman, 2013).

E. faecalis and *E. faecium* are the most important *Enterococcus* spp. causing disease in poultry. *E. durans*, *E. hirae* and *E. cecorum* have been called "species of emerging importance" (Thayer and Waltman, 2013).

Generally, gram-positive cocci can survive for a long time outside of hosts and are relatively resistant against disinfectants.

Vertical transmission of *Staph. aureus* and *Enterococcus* spp. as a consequence of contamination of the eggshell with faeces has been demonstrated. This might also cause reduced hatchability due to an increased number of embryos unable to pip (Fertner et al., 2011).

The bacteria are only capable to cause harm if the defence mechanisms of the host are compromised. This might be a breach of the skin by injuries or after management procedures like desnooding or trimming of toes or beak. Inflammation of damaged respiratory or enteric mucosa might also allow infection. On the other hand, one isolate of *E. faecalis* was also shown to be able to damage the intestinal epithelium on its own (Moore and Gross, 1968). Immune suppressive diseases like infectious bursal disease, infections with haemorrhagic enteritis virus or chicken infectious anaemia can be predisposing factors. The latter can be the underlying cause of gangrenous dermatitis caused by *Staph. aureus*, a condition known as "blue wing disease".

The infection can remain localized at the site of entry, or the bacteria can enter the blood and cause septicaemia. Subsequently, in the subacute or chronic stage, they can infect other organs, most importantly the liver. Additionally, *Staph. aureus* frequently infects the musculoskeletal system and *Streptococcus* spp. and *Enterococcus* spp. the endocardium.

In the case of *Staph. aureus*, several enzymes like hyaluronidase, deoxyribonucleases, lipases or proteases as well as toxins including dermonecrotic toxin, exfoliative toxin and enterotoxins are virulence factors. Coagulase activity is regarded as the main marker of virulence. There is less information about specific virulence factors of *Streptococcus* spp. and *Enterococcus* spp. in poultry.

Certain *E. faecalis* isolates are assumed to be the most important component in the development of amyloid arthropathy, which is frequently accompanied with systemic amyloidosis. The condition can be reproduced in animal studies by intravenous, intraarticular or intraperitoneal infection. However, the route of infection in field cases as well as the factors that distinguish those isolates from *E. faecalis* isolates that do not cause amyloid arthropathy are unknown (Petersen et al., 2008).

Clinical signs

The course of the disease mainly depends on the bacterial isolate and on the underlying causes. Genetic background might play a role in infections with *Staph. aureus* (Cotter and Taylor, 1991) and certainly does so in amyloid arthropathy, which almost exclusively affects brown layers (Petersen et al., 2008).

Besides reduced general condition, especially during septicaemia, acutely infected birds may show lameness with reluctance to walk and inability to stand. In the chronic stage, swollen joints or abscesses might be visible. Plantar abscesses, from which *Staph. aureus* can often be isolated, are also known as bumblefoot. Impaired ability to reach water and feed can cause decreased weight gain or weight loss. Birds may also die peracutely due to septicaemia without first showing clinical signs or only pale or cyanotic combs and wattles. Chicks and poults infected through the navel at the hatchery have a reddened, swollen and inflamed navel.

Morbidity and mortality are usually low and only individual birds are affected; however, in serious cases, mortality can reach 50 % and egg production may drop up to 15 %.

Post mortem lesions

Localized lesions are inflammation of the bones, especially the tibiotarsus or the femur, joints, especially the tibiotarsal or stifle joint, and tendon sheaths or to a lesser extent other organs (Fig. 3). Femoral head necrosis can be due to *Staph. aureus*. The lesions are characterized by accumulation of fibrin. Histologically, the organs are infiltrated by a large number of heterophils and large numbers of coccoid bacteria are visible.

Infection with *Staph. aureus* can cause a greenish discolouration of the liver of turkeys (Fig. 4). If additionally lesions in bones are present, the condition is called green-liver osteomyelitis complex. *Staph. aureus*, *Streptococcus* spp. and *Enterococcus* spp. can cause granulomas in the liver, which are characterized by multifocal necrosis, accumulation of heterophils and thrombosis. Infarcts caused by thrombosis may also be present in spleen, kidney, brain or heart.

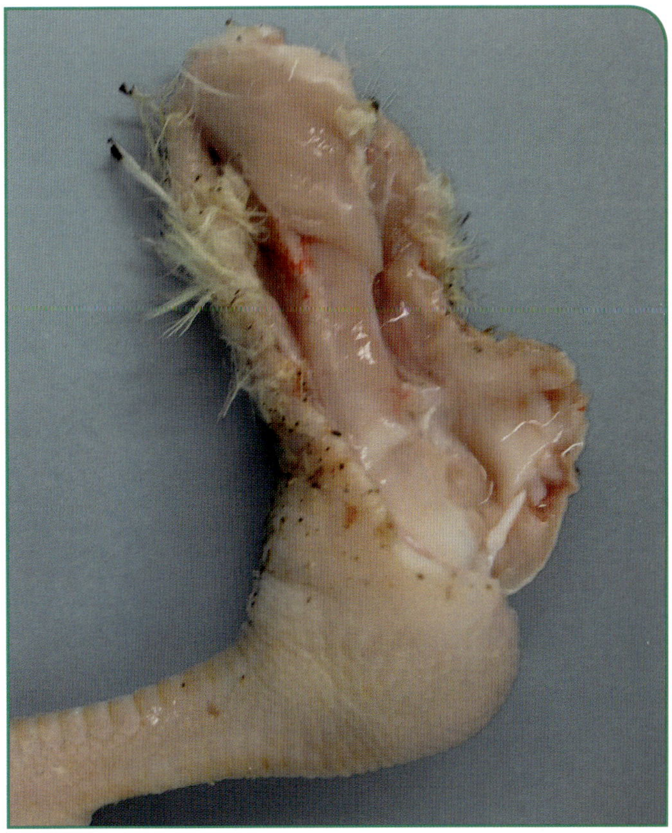

Figure 3. Arthritis and tenosynovitis caused by infection with *Staphylococcus aureus.*

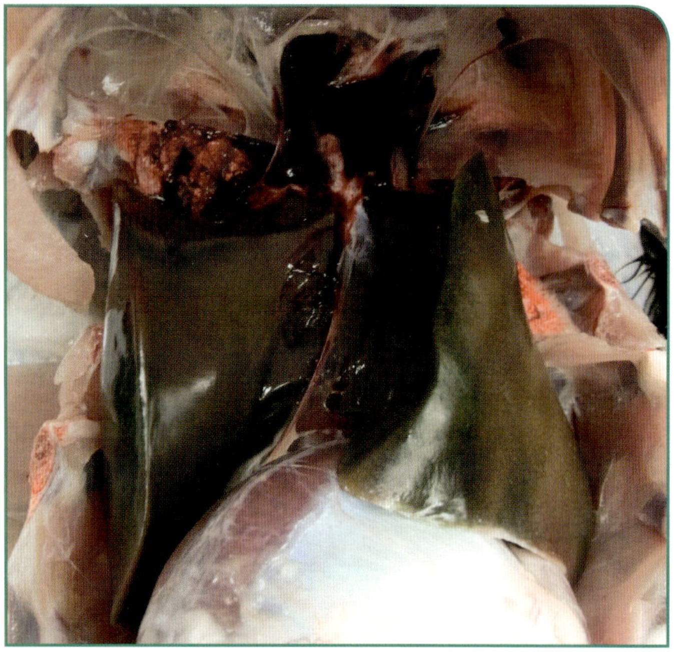

Figure 4. Green discolouration of a turkey liver caused by infection with *Staphylococcus aureus.*

Hearts with endocarditis and especially valvular endocarditis are enlarged, pale and flaccid. Lesions are small, slightly raised, rough and yellowish or tan discoloured (Fig. 5). Histopathologically, accumulations of fibrin, heterophils and bacteria as well as oedema can be seen.

In cases of septicaemia, liver, spleen and kidney are swollen and congested; peritonitis can be present. *Streptococcus* spp. and *Enterococcus* spp. can also cause leptomeningitis and have been associated with encephalomalacia.

Inflammation of the yolk sac is characterized by enlargement, greenish colour, too fluid or too pasty consistency and smell foul (Fig. 6).

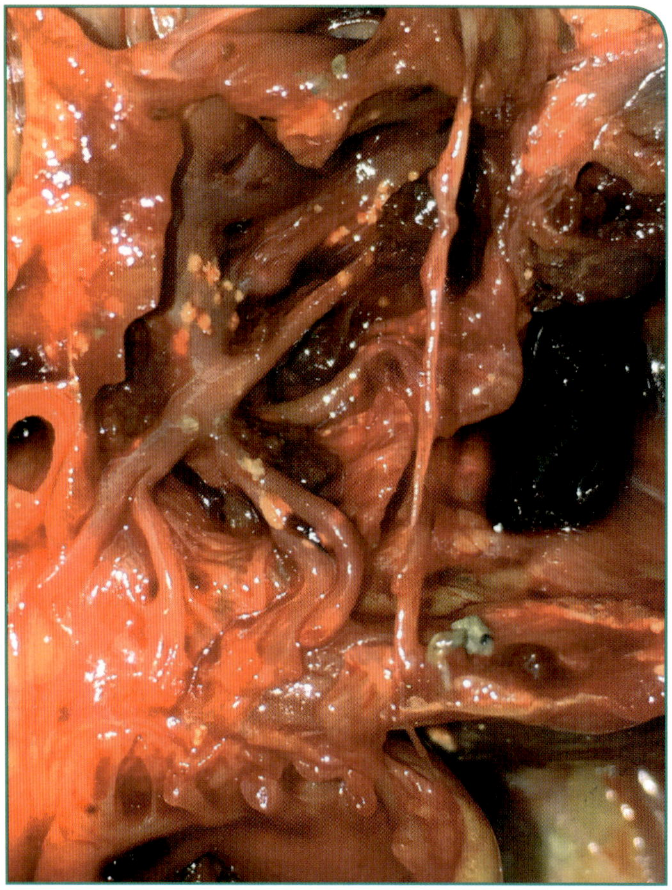

Figure 5. Valvular endocarditis due to infection with *Staphylococcus hyicus.* Image courtesy of Dr. Simone Stoute and Dr. Manuela Crispo (California Animal Health and Food Safety Laboratory System, Turlock branch).

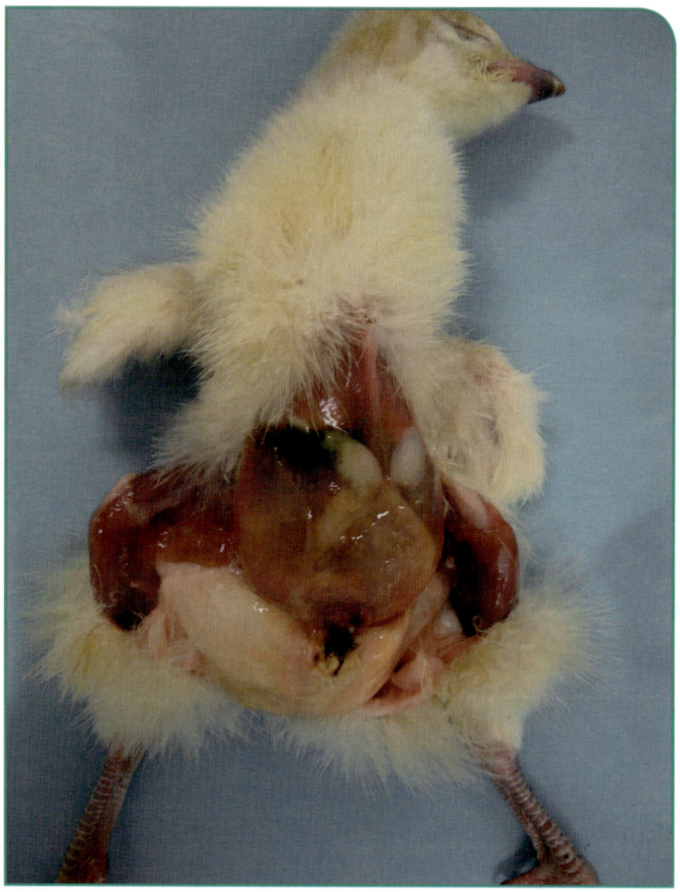

Figure 6. Omphalitis due to infection with *Staphylococcus aureus.*

Diagnostic procedures

Staph. aureus, *Streptococcus* spp. and *Enterococcus* spp. can be easily isolated on blood agar. If samples are taken from sites containing high loads of other bacteria, mannitol salt agar containing 7.5 % NaCl, against which *Staph. aureus* is resistant, or phenylethanol agar, which inhibits growth of gram-negative bacteria, can be used. After incubation under aerobic conditions at 37 °C for 18–24 hours, pinpoint size, circular and smooth colonies are visible. *Staph. aureus* colonies are beta-haemolytic and usually have a yellow to orange colour, which is responsible for the name of the species (Fig. 7). Haemolyisis caused by *Streptococcus* spp. can be variable, while *Enterococcus* spp. do not usually cause haemolysis (Fig. 8) (Andreasen, 2013; Thayer and Waltman, 2013).

As mentioned above, *Staphylococcus* spp. can be differentiated from *Streptococcus* spp. and *Enterococcus* spp. based on their positive catalase reaction and on the clustering of cells. Additionally, some *Enterococcus* spp. isolates can grow on MacConkey agar, while *Streptococcus* spp. cannot.

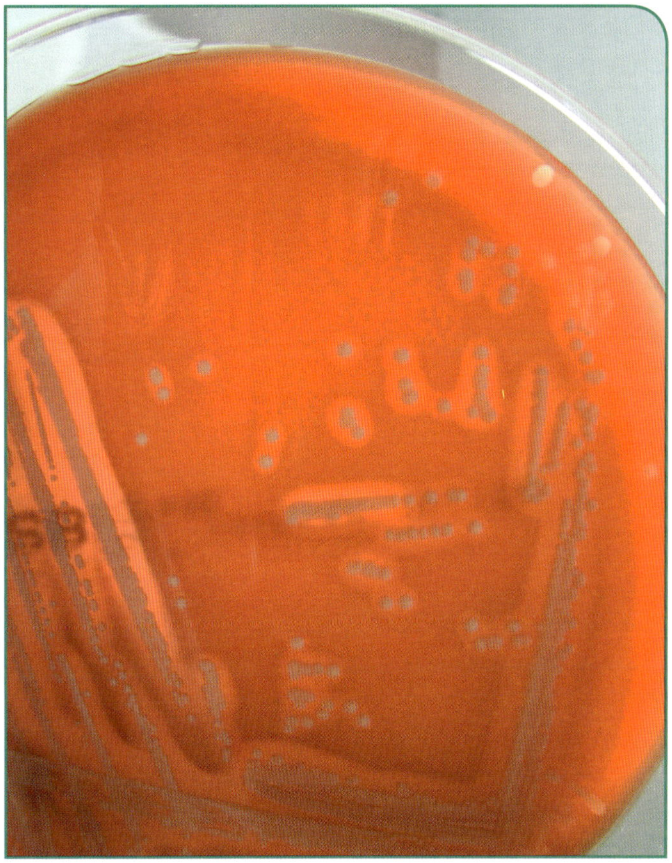

Figure 7. *Staphylococcus aureus* colonies on blood agar. Image courtesy of Dr. Sarah Brüggemann-Schwarze (Institute for Poultry Diseases, Freie Universität Berlin).

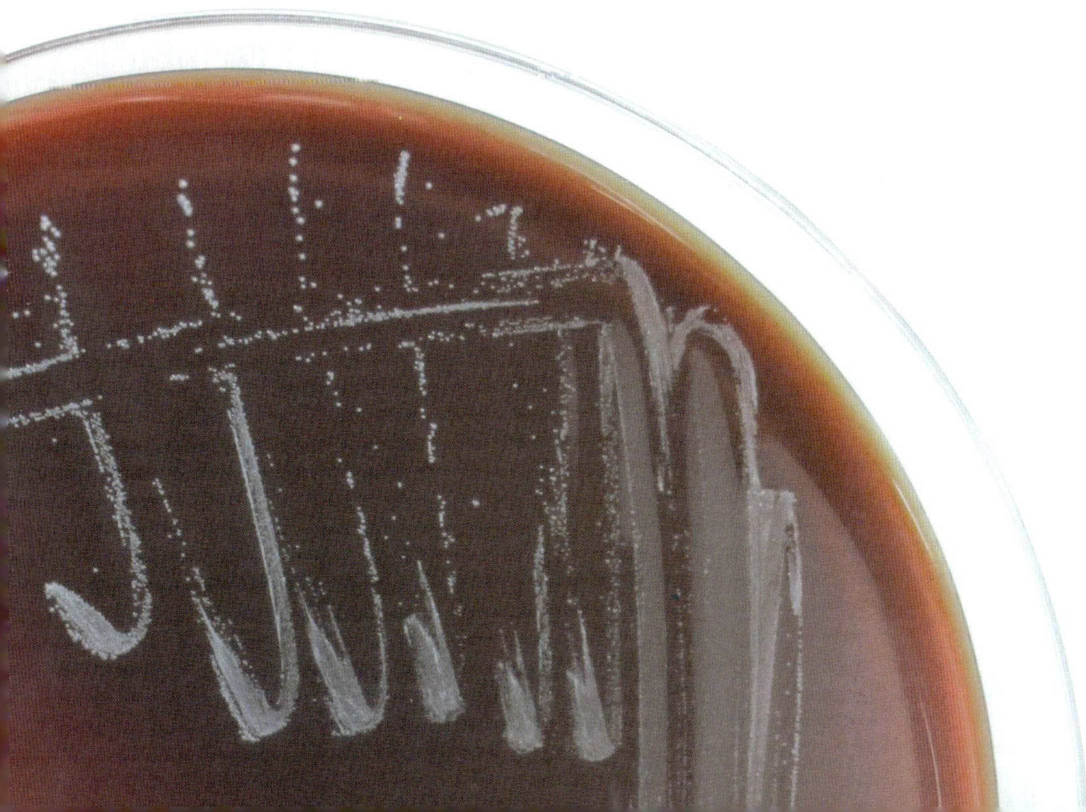

Figure 8. *Streptococcus mutans* colonies on blood agar. Image courtesy of Dr. Sarah Brüggemann-Schwarze (Institute for Poultry Diseases, Freie Universität Berlin).

Definite identification of genus and species usually relies on classical biochemistry or sequencing of the 16 S rRNA gene.

Current commonly used methods for typing *Staph. aureus* are sequence analysis of the protein A gene variable repeat region (spa typing) and multilocus sequence typing (MLST) (Santos-Júnior et al., 2016). MLST can also be used to type *Streptococcus* spp. and *Enterococcus* spp. (Dumke et al., 2015). *Streptococcus* spp. and *Enterococcus* spp. can be typed serologically into Lancefield groups, which is rarely done today.

Several chromogenic media for detection of MRSA or VRE are commercially available (Peltroche-Llacsahuanga et al., 2009; Xu et al., 2016). Phenotypically, resistance against oxacillin or cefoxitin is suggestive of MRSA, but to meet the definition, the presence of a resistance gene, almost always mecA or rarely other variants, needs to be demonstrated (Paterson et al., 2014). VRE, in contrast, are defined phenotypically based on the minimal inhibitory concentration (MIC) of vancomycin, for which one of several resistance genes can be responsible (CLSI, 2016).

Due to the ubiquitous and opportunistic nature of the bacteria, detection of antibodies against them is not considered useful in diagnosis.

Treatment

Treatment is usually effective in cases of septicaemia early during the outbreak. In contrast, the treatment of chronic cases and localized infections is difficult because antibiotics do not often reach the inflamed organs or cannot penetrate into abscesses or granulomas. Furthermore, resistance against antibiotics is common and can be easily acquired by those bacteria. Because of that, if treatment is tried, an antibacterial susceptibility test should be done. Drugs that were helpful in field cases include beta-lactams, tetracyclines, sulphonamides, aminoglycosides and fluoroquinolones.

Control

The most important aspect of prevention of disease due to gram-positive cocci is the prevention of immunosuppressive disease and of management practices impairing the immune system, for example by putting the birds under stress. Management can also help to prevent skin injuries by providing a safe environment free of sharp objects.

Thorough cleaning and disinfection of incubators in hatcheries reduces the infection pressure on the newly hatched birds during the vulnerable phase when their navel is still open.

Inactivated vaccines against *Staph. aureus* were largely ineffective (Thayer and Waltman, 2013). However, application of live, avirulent *Staphylococcus* isolates can act as competitive exclusion due to bacterial interference and have a beneficial effect. Even though this was shown several decades ago in chickens and turkeys (Devriese et al., 1972; Nicoll and Jensen, 1987), no commercial product is on the market. Interestingly, the mechanism of *Staph. epidermidis* strain 115, which gave very good results in turkeys, has been recently elucidated in the search for new antibiotics (Bennallack et al., 2014).

There seems to be no information regarding vaccination of poultry against *Streptococcus* spp. or *Enterococcus* spp.

References

Andreasen CB. Staphylococcosis. In: Diseases of Poultry, DE Swayne, JR Glisson, LR McDougald, LK Nolan, DL Suarez and V. Nair, eds. Ames, Iowa: Wiley-Blackwell. 2013; pp. 971–977.

Bennallack PR, Burt SR, Heder MJ, Robison RA and Griffitts JS. Characterization of a novel plasmid-borne thiopeptide gene cluster in *Staphylococcus epidermidis* strain 115. *Journal of Bacteriology*. 2014; 196, 4344–4350.

Bisgaard M, Bojesen AM, Petersen MR and Christensen H. A major outbreak of *Streptococcus equi* subsp. zooepidemicus infections in free-range chickens is linked to horses. *Avian Diseases*. 56, 561–566.

Caly DL, D'Inca R, Auclair E and Drider D. Alternatives to antibiotics to prevent necrotic enteritis in broiler chickens: a microbiologist's perspective. *Frontiers in Microbiology*. 2015; 6, article 1336.

CLSI. Performance standards for antimicrobial susceptibility testing. 2016.

Cotter PF and Taylor RL. Differential resistance to *Staphylococcus aureus* challenge in two related lines of chickens. *Poultry Science*. 1991; 70, 1357–1361.

Devriese LA, Devos AH and Beumer J. *Staphylococcus aureus* colonization on poultry after experimental spray inoculations. *Avian Diseases*. 1972; 16, 656–665.

Dumke J, Hinse D, Vollmer T, Schulz J, Knabbe C and Dreier J. Potential transmission pathways of *Streptococcus gallolyticus* subsp. gallolyticus. *PLoS ONE*. 2015; 10: e0126507.

Fertner ME, Olsen RH, Bisgaard M and Christensen H. Transmission and genetic diversity of *Enterococcus faecalis* among layer chickens during hatch. *Acta Veterinaria Scandinavica*. 2011; 53, 56.

Franz CMAP, Huch M, Abriouel H, Holzapfel W and Gálvez A. Enterococci as probiotics and their implications in food safety. *International Journal of Food Microbiology*. 2011; 151, 125–140.

Moore WE and Gross WB. Liver granulomas of turkeys – causative agents and mechanism of infection. *Avian Diseases*. 1968; 12, 417–422.

Nicoll TR and Jensen MM. Staphylococcosis of turkeys. 5. Large-scale control programs using bacterial interference. *Avian Diseases*. 1987; 31, 85–88.

Paterson GK, Harrison EM and Holmes MA. The emergence of mecC methicillin-resistant *Staphylococcus aureus*. *Trends in Microbiology*. 2014; 22, 42–47.

Peltroche-Llacsahuanga H, Top J, Weber-Heynemann J, Lütticken R and Haase G. Comparison of two chromogenic media for selective isolation of vancomycin-resistant enterococci from stool specimens. *Journal of Clinical Microbiology*. 2009; 47, 4113–4116.

Petersen A, Chadfield MS, Christensen JP, Christensen H and Bisgaard M. Characterization of small-colony variants of *Enterococcus faecalis* isolated from chickens with amyloid arthropathy. *Journal of Clinical Microbiology*. 2008; 46, 2686–2691.

Santos-Júnior CD, Veríssimo A and Costa J. The recombination dynamics of *Staphylococcus aureus* inferred from spA gene. *BMC Microbiology*. 2016; 16, 143.

Shi D, Fang D, Hu X, Li A, Lv L, Guo J, Chen Y, Wu W, Guo F and Li L. Draft genome sequence of *Staphylococcus gallinarum* DSM 20610T, originally isolated from the skin of a chicken. *Genome Announcements*. 2015; 3, e00580-15.

Thayer SG and Waltman WD. Streptococcus and Enterococcus. In: Diseases of Poultry, DE Swayne, JR Glisson, LR McDougald, LK Nolan, DL Suarez and V Nair, eds. Ames, Iowa: Wiley-Blackwell. 2013; pp. 977–985.

Xu Z, Hou Y, Peters BM, Chen D, Li B, Li L and Shirtliff ME. Chromogenic media for MRSA diagnostics. *Molecular Biology Reports*. 2016; 1–8.

Published by Servet editorial - Grupo Asís Biomedia S.L.